# DISCOVER NUTRITIONAL THERAPY

# DISCOVER
# NUTRITIONAL
# THERAPY

## PATRICIA QUINN

Ulysses Press ⚏ Berkeley, CA

1998

Published by: Ulysses Press
P.O. Box 3440
Berkeley, CA 94703-3440

Library of Congress Catalog Card Number: 98-84067

ISBN: 1-56975-135-8

Printed in Canada by Transcontinental Printing

First published as *Healing with Nutritional Therapy,* Gill & Macmillan, 1998

10 9 8 7 6 5 4 3 2 1

Editorial: Steven Schwartz, Lily Chou, Marguerite Clipper
Typesetter: David Wells
Cover Design: B & L Design
Indexer: Sayre Van Young

Distributed in the United States by Publishers Group West and in Canada by Raincoast Books

This book has been written and published strictly for informational purposes, and in no way should it be used as a substitute for consultation with your medical doctor or other health care professional. All facts in this book came from medical files, clinical journals, scientific publications, personal interviews, published trade books, self-published materials by experts, magazine articles, and the personal-practice experiences of the authorities quoted or sources cited. You should not consider educational material herein to be the practice of medicine or to replace consultation with a physician or other medical practitioner. The author and publisher are providing you with information in this work so that you can have the knowledge and can choose, at your own risk, to act on that knowledge. The author and publisher also urge all readers to be aware of their health status and to consult health professionals before beginning any health program, including changes in dietary habits.

# TABLE OF CONTENTS

# WHAT IS NUTRITIONAL THERAPY?

Nutritional therapy is a system of healing based on the belief that food as nature intended provides the medicine we need to obtain and maintain a state of health: our food is our medicine and our medicine is our food. Although some health problems require specific medication, many conditions can be relieved effectively with nutritional therapy. These include disorders ranging from chronic fatigue, energy loss, insomnia and depression to backache, skin complaints, asthma and headaches. Nutritional therapy will also benefit you if you have no specific illness, but want to maintain a state of optimum health. It is safe for babies and children as well as adults, and the change of eating patterns that is typically prescribed usually has far fewer side effects than synthetic medicines.

Nutritional therapy is a holistic discipline; nutrition as the key to good health is the all-embracing fundamental principle used since the time of the famous Greek doctor and founder of western medicine, Hippocrates, to help people of all ages to stay at their personal peak of energy and vitality. Today, new insights of food scientists play a significant role in the practice of nutritional therapy as preventative medicine.

During the last fifty years many wonderful breakthroughs have improved our understanding of the role of food in our lives. But at the same time, many of us are realizing that food is the cornerstone which, in our modern lifestyle, has been rejected by the builder.

The speed at which we live and work — the pressure of the deadline — pushes us into a fast-eating culture, where quality of food becomes secondary. Eating on the job, on the run, under pressure, denies us the experience, the purpose and the role of food. Eventually it denies us our very lifestyle. Modern supermarkets are stocked with many instant meals, but more often than not, these meals are far lower in nutritional value than those prepared at home with fresh organically grown ingredients.

For all the benefits agribusiness has brought the people of the Western world, the disadvantages of the modern food industry include extensive use of chemicals in food production. There is also a loss of the vitality intrinsic in newly harvested food because many products are transported vast distances before they reach their destination. Of course, this is the case with many of the so-called "fresh" foods on our supermarket shelves, as well as with those dishes that have been pre-cooked and packaged before reaching the supermarkets.

Lifestyle and nutrition are intimately linked, and our lifestyle defines itself partly from the tradition of the country we live in and partly from our attitudes. How do you really want to live? Given the choice, would you prefer to eat well every day, to exercise, to breathe clean air as often as possible, to drink a reasonable amount of water in order to keep your bloodstream clean and able to wash out toxins? This choice is available to all of us, but to exercise it we need to understand the impact on our well-being of different foods and learn from direct experience what kind of eating pattern best suits our lifestyle.

## WHAT IS HEALTH?

In a dynamic and good state of health, our mental, emotional, physical and spiritual components all live in harmony with each other. For a wider comprehension of health, it is interesting to look at the issue of "healthiness" not only from the Western but also from the Eastern viewpoint. The ancient systems of Chinese and Indian medicine go back more than 5,000 years. These cultures used — and continue to use — whole plants in their treatment, whereas orthodox medicine uses extracts from plants which are often then replicated by synthetic products.

The two systems of medicine diverge at the point of prevention. Eastern practices include the preventative care of the whole person as a primary aim — to maintain good health. The formula for good health is:

- life force

- good-quality blood

- proper nourishment

Our daily diet will make good-quality blood, which in turn promotes the flow of healthy energy. We need to ask ourselves daily questions. What is my physical health like today? Do I have a sense of well-being? Do I have plenty of energy? Do I sleep and eat well? How we feel each day is built upon our past actions, our past dietary practices, whether we have had physical exercise, whether we have been mentally active, and on our general attitude towards life.

## TIREDNESS VERSUS FATIGUE

Fatigue is very prevalent in the present day. The healthy person who uses his or her entire body in the ways described above during each day will feel tired — the pleasant feeling of having worked hard. This individual's body will be able to relax completely and recuperate at the end of the day. This is not fatigue — it is the body's natural need for rest. It is during rest and recuperation that the body cleanses itself of all the toxins that build up during activity. If the body is not given a chance to self-cleanse, a state of fatigue will become persistent. When it becomes chronic, fatigue may indicate underlying problems, such as infection, immune system weaknesses, glandular problems or lymphatic congestion, as the body's systems become clogged by waste.

## WHAT IS ILLNESS?

Illness develops in four stages:

- tiredness, changing to fatigue — no amount of rest seems adequate

- irritability

- symptoms

- illness

The Eastern approach to health divides the causes of illness into two: those that come from within and those that come from without. Those from within are mostly products of our lifestyle, traditions and beliefs. The ways we can be affected from within are as follows:

- excess of emotions, even positive ones such as joy, can affect the heart

- excess of anger can affect the liver

- excess of sadness damages the appetite, the stomach, spleen or pancreas

- excessive grief can affect the lungs

- shock, fear, surprise or fright can affect the kidneys

Part of the process of nutritional therapy is to help us restore the proper balance, to bring about the harmony we lack.

## THE "FOUR DOCTORS"

The basic needs of our physical bodies to eliminate toxic waste, as described above, are being denied to us by the life we lead in modern Western society. What we require to attend to these basic needs I call the "four doctors":

1. sunlight and fresh air

2. proper exercise and sufficient rest

3. good food

4. pure water

While our ancestors lived mainly outdoor lives, we tend to live largely indoors, denying ourselves the most pivotal requirement: light. Our whole body depends on the reception of light in order to carry out vital functions — the regulation of the appetite, our patterns of sleeping and waking, aspects of our behavior and the health of our nervous system. Fresh air is necessary for us to exchange the toxins and pollutants in the body with at least an equal amount of air. Otherwise, we develop acute respiratory problems from overload; our cities do not have sufficient trees to breathe back oxygen into our environment. Trees act as "lungs" by filling the air with life-giving oxygen.

Water is the greatest treat for the body. It is the river that carries all the nutrients around the body to the brain, and to every single cell in the body. The brain is the first place to suffer dehydration — it then becomes difficult to think or make appropriate decisions. In recent studies, it was found that water more than food helped give long-distance walkers the energy to finish. Likewise, those driving long distances need a snack as well as a break of fifteen minutes or so in order to maintain their concentration on the road. In both of these examples, the simple remedies prevented emotional and psychological imbalance, which drains the body of its energy supply and causes fatigue.

## THE ROLE OF FOOD IN OUR LIVES

By experimenting with the effects of different foods, many people find they also revise old beliefs about the role of food in their lives. Nutritional therapy is not just about eating different types of food — it is also about increasing your awareness of how you eat and of where the food you eat comes from, of how you store and prepare it, and of how you perceive yourself and your place in the web of life. The benefits of nutritional therapy are sometimes immediate, but its study is timeless and its effects can bring about long-lasting changes in your attitude to life.

Recently, Dr. Henry Dreher — author of *The Immune Power Personality* — reminded us of certain characteristics we can all develop which increase our ability to be healthy. These characteristics include

- having the ability to recognize when the body is signalling to us that it is in pain or feeling tired

- identifying emotions such as anger or sadness

- connecting these states to food we have recently eaten and so learning to identify the effects different foods have on us

- developing a sense of control over our health and over the quality of our lives, because the way we live — as well as the way we eat — is part of the way we nourish ourselves

Nutritional therapy helps us consider our human immunity in the context of a rapidly changing environment by deepening our understanding of the constant ebb and flow between ourselves and our outer world. Our immunity is part of the entire picture — a relationship between our own evolving and our world. "Whole body" immunity concerns all aspects of life: ensuring that the physical body has the correct nutrition and appropriate healing therapies, enjoying good emotional health by nurturing the feelings, learning to make choices from a position of unbiased awareness and not from the "victim" or "martyr" approach.

Nutritional therapy requires us to acknowledge that we are body, soul, mind and emotion. Accordingly, it incorporates all these aspects of our lives, with the objective of maintaining a healthy mind and soul as well as a healthy body, developing an open-minded outlook and a positive attitude to ourselves, and learning to see any causes of stress in our lives as challenges rather than threats.

# 2

# THE HISTORY OF NUTRITIONAL HEALING

A monk asked, "Is there anything more miraculous than the wonders of Nature?" The master replied, "Yes — your appreciation of the wonders of Nature."

In Ancient Greece, the two philosophies of medicine and healing were under the patronage of two different gods. The doctors worked under the patronage of Asclepius, god of medicine, while Asclepius's beautiful daughter Hygeia (goddess of health, whose name is the origin of the word *hygiene*) was the patron of healers. In around 400 B.C., Hippocrates was writing his memoirs on the medicinal uses of herbs, spices and food. At about the same time, and of equal importance, the man known as the father of botany, Theophrastus, was recording the extensive botanical knowledge of the day and the wide variety of uses herbs and spices were found to have.

Later, when the Romans occupied Britain in the first century A.D., they looked after the medical needs of their soldiers with a variety of herbs and spices. In fact, they brought 400 herbs with them to Britain, which they planted and harvested. These new herbs added to an already extensive body of knowledge that had been handed down from generation to generation by the Druids.

In the sixth century, the religious orders began to found their monasteries. They grew their herbs in kitchen gardens, while the hospitals filled their gardens with herbs to feed the sick. Spices were, of course, as highly prized as gold, because they were so difficult to get from the Orient and the Near East. There was a widely held traditional belief among the ordinary people, who in their own kitchens were cooking vegetables, grains, fruit and meats, that these spices also held the elements necessary to heal disease.

## James Lind's Cure for Scurvy

In the year 1747, James Lind, who was the surgeon's mate on the HMS *Salisbury*, made the brilliant discovery that two oranges and one lemon eaten daily over a six-day period completely reversed the symptoms of scurvy (a vitamin C deficiency that caused widespread weakness, disease and death among sailors). Lind did not know anything about vitamins, but his remedy was extremely effective. He had used food as medicine. Yet it was only in 1795 that the British admiralty put his simple preventative medicine into action. From 1795, an ounce of lemon juice per day wiped out scurvy in the English Merchant Navy. Many more years were to pass, however, before this simple preventative measure was extended to the Royal Navy.

## The Effects of Refined Foods

During the early nineteenth century, further experiments with food proved that the fat, carbohydrate and protein content of food — while essential for life — were not sufficient to support growth, nor for the healthy development of the eyes. When the steel roller mill was introduced in 1830, white flour became cheaper and more widely available. Until then, the people of Europe had eaten a wide variety of fruits, vegetables, grains, herbs and, recently, spices. The change in diet to refined white flour, white rice and white sugar caused widespread vitamin deficiency. Serious illnesses such as beriberi became known wherever these foods spread.

In the West Indies, a young Dutch physician called Christiaan Eijkman was assigned in 1886 to study beriberi. He observed that the chickens in the laboratory chicken yard were suffering from a disease that paralleled all the symptoms of beriberi. He discovered through a process of observation and inquiry that the regular diet of the patients in the military hospital was white rice. Most of the chickens were fed the leftovers. When a new cook took over he refused to feed the patients anything other than whole grain unpolished rice. With this change both the patients and the chickens revived and went on to become very healthy.

Eijkman then did a widespread study of Dutch West Indies prisoners. He found that beriberi was 300 times more prevalent in prisoners where polished (white) rice rather than unpolished rice was the staple diet. He concluded that the bran of the rice contained a substance or nutrient necessary for health.

## NATUROPATHIC MEDICINE

Right up to the present day, the debate continues about the very nature of health. But the most basic tenet of all healing — whether mental, emotional, physical, spiritual, chemical, or all these things — is that nature heals. This has been the central theme of naturopathic medicine, the precursor to nutritional therapy.

A great surge in natural therapies occurred in the nineteenth century in Europe and America, and written legacies of enormous value were produced by naturopaths such as Vincent Priessnitz, Jethro Kloss, Sebastian Kneipp and J. H. Kellogg. While some physicians chose to specialize in naturopathic medicine, others throughout the world worked within their own sphere of medicine, developing, expanding and increasing their understanding of nutrition within the context of a particular discipline. While working with the principle that outside intervention is necessary on one hand and nature works towards healing on the other, the naturopath's approach maintains that the constant effort of the body's life force is always in the direction of self-cleansing, self-repair and positive health. According to this approach, every cell in the body is imbued with an instinct of self-preservation sustained by an inherent force known as "the vital force of life."

## THE DISCOVERY OF VITAMINS

In 1911, the Polish scientist Casimir Funk proposed the theory that there were anti-scurvy, anti-beriberi, anti-pellagra and anti-rickets factors in food. He called these food factors "vitamins" (from the Latin *vita*, meaning "life"). Then Albert Szent-Györgyi of Budapest gave the crystalline substance he had isolated from the adrenal gland of the ox to the English sugar chemist W. N. Haworth, who found its structural formula. It was ascorbic acid — the acidic substance that prevents scurvy! In 1937, these two men each received a Nobel prize for their work in finally finding the substance which in 1747 James Lind had proven, through a simple test with oranges and lemons, to save people's lives at sea. Extensive research into vitamins in subsequent decades has established that we need a balanced intake of vitamins A, B, C, D and E to maintain health. Lists of foods containing these vitamins are included in Appendix One (see page 92).

## THE DISCOVERY OF MINERALS

The study of minerals in food began in the 1940s — until that time, only iodine and iron were known and understood to be essential to life. Since the 1940s, numerous major discoveries have been made — we now know of a whole range of minerals essential to good health, such as zinc, iodine and potassium. By identifying vitamin and mineral imbalances, today's doctors can reverse many serious illnesses that were previously undiagnosable.

## THE BIRTH OF NUTRITIONAL MEDICINE

In 1968, Dr. Linus Pauling defined orthomolecular medicine, with particular reference to psychiatry as a way of achieving and preserving mental health by varying the concentrations in the human body of substances that are normally present, such as vitamins. This definition was the crystallization of what we now know as nutritional medicine. Dr. Pauling won the Nobel Prize for Chemistry in 1954, and the Nobel Prize for Peace in 1963. His pioneering work gave medicine a new impetus. Until his research was recognized, nutrition and medicine had become polarized as separate professions.

In recent decades, a succession of nutritional breakthroughs all over the world has gradually brought new evidence to light about the properties in food that are essential to good health. The Hippocratic school, which treated disease with diet, fasting, hydrotherapy, exercise and spinal manipulation, may yet become recognized once more as a cornerstone of medical practice.

## LOCAL FOOD

The gastronomic life of a country used to be based primarily on climate and geographical position, which suggests there may have been some uniformity in eating patterns among people who lived along particular latitudes and in similar land-masses. But occupation by peoples with other eating habits can radically alter the native diet. This is how viniculture superseded beer and apple brewing in Europe following the Roman occupation of England and France. But national preferences for foods die hard, because they are deeply associated with the culture, not just the dinner plate.

## The Impact of Industrialization on Diet

The impact of industrialization, however, particularly in the sphere of agriculture, and the new wave of technology, have contributed to a loss of awareness about our local dietary heritage. In England, the movement from a rural and agricultural society to an urban industrial society in the nineteenth century had devastating effects on workers' diets. Widespread malnutrition was dealt with at that time through the mass production and distribution of basic foodstuffs by religious institutions, in particular the Quaker foundations and families such as Fry and Cadbury. The era of processed food was about to dawn. And it was the answer to a definite demand.

At first, this kind of food relieved malnutrition and susceptibility to contagious diseases, so how is it today that processed food adds to our health problems? That processed food is directly linked with obesity, diabetes, heart disease and cancer is irrefutable. But there are many additional contributing factors. For example, most of us exercise far less than we did in the centuries before the invention of the automobile. Prior to the revolution in transport and technology the pace of life was far slower than it is now, and before the introduction of intensive farming techniques processed foods were typically combined with locally grown produce.

Nutritional analysts have observed that when a country industrializes slowly, its people have maintained their cultural heritage in general and their food heritage in particular. Southern France, Italy and Spain, the coast of the Middle East and the Greek islands all share the now revered "Mediterranean Diet." They still adhere to their regional preferences but have in common with other coast-dwelling peoples, such as the Scandinavians and Japanese, access to certain very beneficial sea foods. By comparison, the people of countries that have industrialized rapidly, such as England and, more recently, Japan (where these changes are beginning to make detrimental inroads on the benefits of the traditional diet) and parts of China, quickly lose touch with their food heritage. Time becomes a precious commodity, and as fewer people work on the land, knowledge of the qualities in local food diminishes while less nutritious imported food products become fashionable. For example, processed cereals are now a feature of most English households, yet these are both more expensive and less nutritious than a simple dish such as porridge with dried fruits. Similarly, in many parts of Japan, refined white bread has replaced a more nutritious traditional breakfast of egg, rice and bean curd.

### THE EFFECTS OF INTENSIVE AGRICULTURE

Overall, we can see that while research into the nutrients of food has made a huge contribution to our knowledge during the course of the twentieth century, at the same time loss of local knowledge — combined with intensive use of artificial fertilizers in food cultivation and the export of basic foodstuffs on a massive scale — have contributed to a deterioration in our overall health. However, once you understand the central significance of food in your life, you can make several simple adjustments to your eating patterns to ensure that you receive the nutrients you need. You do not have to be a scientist to benefit from the insights of nutritional therapy; the next section of this book will show how many of the precepts of nutritional therapy are based on simple self-awareness, self-observation and common sense.

# 3

# ESSENTIAL NUTRIENTS

The body requires a certain daily intake of nutrients in the form of carbohydrates, fats, minerals, proteins, vitamins and water. If your body is deficient in any of these, illness will result. Sometimes the illness may be caused by a clear absence of the appropriate nutrient in your diet; in other instances the deficiency may arise because of the body's inability to absorb a particular nutrient properly. In these cases, an alternative way of providing the nutrient must be found.

## CARBOHYDRATES

Carbohydrates are the body's major source of energy, and are made up of sugars, starch and fiber. They are also needed to metabolize proteins for body tissue repair and to run the central nervous system. Unrefined carbohydrates include all grains, such as rice, wheat, oats, barley and millet. They lose their nutritional value through refinement (e.g. white bread, white rice and white sugar) and provide only "empty" calories.

Lack of carbohydrates leads to listlessness, fatigue and nausea. Getting too many refined carbohydrates leads to obesity, tooth decay, high blood pressure, heart disease and diabetes.

## FATS

Fats are needed for energy and to create layers of protective tissue in the body. They provide over twice as much energy, weight for weight, as carbohydrates and proteins, so comparatively little fat is needed in the average diet.

Fats are divided into three categories: saturated, monounsaturated and polyunsaturated. Saturated fats are found mainly in food from animal sources, including whole milk, cheese, eggs, cream and butter. These saturated fats also contain high amounts of cholesterol.

Monounsaturated and polyunsaturated fats are found mainly in vegetable oils and soft margarines. They contain no cholesterol. Polyunsaturated fats also contain three essential acids: linoleic acid, oleic acid and arachidonic acid. Linoleic acid enables the body to synthesize other fats from food. It is also thought to help reduce the level of cholesterol in the blood.

Too much fat can lead to obesity, which increases the risk of diabetes, high blood pressure, arthritis and gallbladder disease.

## FOLIC ACID

Folic acid is one of the B vitamins (see below). It helps in the formation of RNA and DNA, and in the breakdown of proteins into amino acids. It is especially important in the early months of pregnancy. Lack of folic acid leads to poor growth, gastrointestinal problems and anemia.

## MINERALS

Minerals are vital for cell growth and repair and the self-regulation of the body. The macro-minerals (calcium, phosphorus, magnesium, sodium, potassium and chloride) are needed in quantities of 100 mg or more per day. The micro-minerals (iron, iodine and zinc) are needed in far smaller quantities. A balance of minerals is very important, as they often work in conjunction with each other.

### CALCIUM

Calcium is essential for the healthy growth of bones, teeth, nails and hair, for the functioning of the nervous system, and for maintenance of muscular contractions. It is present in almonds, almond spreads, fish, molasses, sunflower seeds, sunflower seed spread, green vegetables, kelp, sea vegetables such as kombu, wakame, dulse and hijiki, sesame seeds, tahini (sesame spread), tofu, cottage cheese, cheddar cheese, goat's milk, goat cheese and yogurt, sheep's milk, sheep cheese and feta cheese, ricotta cheese and natural yogurt. Lack of calcium can lead to muscular problems, brittle bones and tooth decay. It can also cause insomnia and nervous exhaustion.

### CHLORIDE

Chloride is needed with sodium and potassium to regulate the body's fluids. It helps in the formation of gastric juices in the stomach for the effective digestion of proteins. Lack of chloride can lead to an imbalance of sodium in the body.

### IODINE

Iodine is necessary for the formation and healthy functioning of two hormones in the thyroid gland that regulate metabolism and protein synthesis. Lack of iodine can lead to obesity, swelling and listlessness.

*IRON*

Iron is necessary for the formation of hemoglobin in red blood cells, which transport oxygen from the lungs throughout the body. To work effectively, iron needs to be balanced with a trace of copper and vitamin C. Lack of iron leads to anemia and fatigue.

*MAGNESIUM*

Magnesium combines with calcium and phosphorus to provide healthy functioning of the skeletal and nervous systems. Lack of magnesium leads to muscular weakness and delirium.

*PHOSPHORUS*

Phosphorus combines with calcium for the healthy formation of bones and teeth, and assists in the body's release of energy.

*POTASSIUM*

Potassium works with sodium to regulate the body's fluids, particularly in the muscle cells and the blood. Lack of potassium can lead to impaired neuromuscular functioning and even to heart attacks.

*SODIUM*

Sodium regulates the body's fluid balance and monitors the passage of nutrients into, and waste out of, the cells. Too much sodium causes fluid retention and high blood pressure.

*SULPHUR*

Sulphur constitutes 0.05 percent of the earth's crust. It is a constituent of all proteins and is present in a number of amino acids. It is also found in vitamin D, thiamine and biotin. It is present in the nails, skin, joints and hair. Sulphur can be obtained from a wide range of sources, some of which include eggs, nuts, garlic, poultry, meat, fish, milk, cheese, mustard and cress, pears, apricots and oatmeal.

## ZINC

Zinc is essential for the growth and repair of tissues, for protein synthesis and for the body's immune system. Lack of zinc causes fatigue, low resistance to infection and stunted sexual maturity.

## PROTEINS

Proteins are essential for the formation, growth and repair of all body cells, and for the functioning of the enzymes, hormones and antibodies that regulate and control our bodies. Proteins are made up of amino acids. There are about twenty amino acids, eight of which are present in protein-containing foods. The rest are synthesized by the body from these eight. Foods that contain all of the eight essential amino acids are called complete proteins; foods that contain only a few are referred to as incomplete proteins.

Dairy products, meat, eggs and fish all contain complete protein. Vegetable proteins such as peas, beans and lentils, grains and vegetables are called incomplete proteins because they do not contain the full spectrum of essential building blocks, or essential amino acids. However, many traditional peoples combine incomplete, non-meat foods in a way that comfortably fulfills our minds' and bodies' protein requirements, without the detrimental effects that can accompany a meat-rich diet. In 1971, food writer Frances Moore Lappé introduced the idea of complementary proteins to modern readers with her book *Diet for a Small Planet*, which is now regarded as a classic.

Lack of protein leads to a decrease in the metabolic process and, in extreme cases of deprivation, eventually to starvation.

**VITAMINS**

Vitamins are usually needed only in tiny quantities, but they are crucial to the healthy functioning of the body. Vitamins are classified in six groups: A, B, C, D, E and K. Vitamins in groups B and C are water-soluble, which means they must be taken regularly because the body cannot store them for a long period of time. Vitamins in groups A, D, E and K are fat-soluble and last longer.

### VITAMIN A (RETINOL)

Vitamin A helps in cell differentiation. It is also needed for healthy skin and mucous membranes and for good night vision. Lack of vitamin A leads to softening of the bones and teeth, dry skin and night blindness.

### VITAMIN B

The major function of the B vitamins is to break down food into simple sugar molecules for energy and to form new red blood cells. The B vitamins are also important for the healthy functioning of the brain, nervous and circulatory systems, and for healthy hair, skin and eyes. B vitamins work most effectively in conjunction with each other.

### VITAMIN $B_1$ (THIAMINE)

Vitamin $B_1$ breaks down carbohydrates for energy. It also assists the functioning of the brain, nerves and muscles. Lack of vitamin $B_1$ leads to constipation and abdominal pains, and in extreme cases to beriberi.

### VITAMIN $B_2$ (RIBOFLAVIN)

Vitamin $B_2$ breaks down fats, carbohydrates and proteins for energy. It is easily destroyed by exposure to light. Lack of vitamin $B_2$ leads to mouth and throat infections and eye fatigue. Riboflavin deficiency is common in nonmilk drinkers.

## VITAMIN B₃ (NIACIN)

Vitamin $B_3$ breaks down fats, carbohydrates and proteins for energy. Lack of vitamin $B_3$ leads to digestive disorders, a sore, swollen tongue and impairment of growth in children.

## VITAMIN B₆ (PYRIDOXINE)

Vitamin $B_6$ breaks down proteins into amino acids for the formation of red blood cells and hormones. Lack of vitamin $B_6$ leads to anemia, nervous disorders and fatigue.

## VITAMIN B₁₂ (COBALAMIN)

Vitamin $B_{12}$ is essential for the formation of red blood cells and for synthesizing RNA and DNA. It is also essential for the healthy functioning of the nervous system. Dairy products are a rich source of vitamin $B_{12}$. Lack of vitamin $B_{12}$ leads to serious anemia.

## VITAMIN C (ASCORBIC ACID)

Vitamin C is essential for the formation of antibodies and for aiding recovery after an infection or illness. It helps to form collagen, which is needed for the body's connective tissue. It is also needed for the absorption of iron and for producing hemoglobin and adrenaline. Lack of vitamin C leads to bleeding gums, poor teeth, low resistance to disease and slow recovery from illness.

## VITAMIN D (CALCIFEROL)

Vitamin D helps the body to absorb and regulate its intake of calcium and phosphorus, and is needed for strong bones, teeth and gums. It is absorbed through sunlight as well as food. Lack of vitamin D causes softening of the bones and, in severe cases, rickets.

## *VITAMIN E (TOCOPHEROL)*

Vitamin E protects vitamin A and the unsaturated fats in the body from harmful oxidation. It also assists in healing after injury or illness. Lack of vitamin E causes muscular wasting, abnormal fat deposits and abnormal red blood cells.

## *VITAMIN K (PHYTOMENADIONE)*

Vitamin K is essential for blood clotting. Lack of vitamin K can lead to internal and external bleeding.

## EIGHT ESSENTIAL ELEMENTS

Of the nutrients listed above, there are seven elements essential for life. These are vitamins A, B, C and D, iodine, sulphur and iron. Citric acid is another element essential for life. It is a constituent of the metabolic pathway of the Krebs cycle, which produces energy in the body. (The Krebs cycle is a very important part of the digestive system.) Never has there been so much demand for these substances as supplements, because never before in human history has our food been cultivated with such artificial and damaging methods.

4

# FOODS THAT HARM,
# FOODS THAT HEAL

If you suffer from a particular complaint or imbalance — for example, if you are deficient in a particular mineral, or if you have difficulty digesting certain kinds of food — you will need to be given herbal or mineral supplements by your nutritional therapist. But there are basic guidelines for healthy eating that apply to all of us. Once you have become aware of what foods harm and what foods heal, and revised your eating patterns accordingly, you will have taken a major step toward increased well-being.

## FOODS THAT HARM

Foods that are detrimental to health, and specifically to the healthy functioning of the thyroid gland, include refined white flour, white sugar, salty foods such as chips and fries, foods with a high salt content, processed meats such as hot dogs and sausage, and caffeine-rich foods such as tea, coffee and chocolate.

### DISTINGUISHING BETWEEN NATURAL AND REFINED SUGAR

The word sugar has two meanings. Sugar as we have known it since the middle of the nineteenth century refers to white sugar, extracted from sugar cane or beets, and brown sugar, extracted from molasses. If we rely too heavily on refined foods that contain these sugars, we bypass the needs of our digestive system, which is designed to work efficiently to break down whole foods, extracting the goodness from them for our bodies.

When sugar is consumed in its refined form (as in sweets, drinks, cakes and other processed foods made with white or brown sugar) it does not nourish us — it robs us. Our stores of B vitamins and our all-important bone-building minerals start to leak out from their storage sites. Binge eating can also develop, as the sugar leaves a "hunger gap," caused by the lack of nutrients.

We may also become addicted to sugar. If eating one small piece of chocolate, cake or cookie does not satisfy but leads instead to an endless craving, this indicates the strong possibility of addiction. To break the cycle, it is better to reduce your intake of refined sugar gradually than to cut it out of your diet completely. At the same time, start to introduce foods containing natural sugar into your diet (see below).

### PROBLEMS ASSOCIATED WITH EXCESSIVE SUGAR INTAKE

The first victims of excessive sugar intake are our teeth, which suffer from loss of calcium, attacks from bacteria and dental caries. Other problems associated with too much refined sugar include low blood sugar and diabetes; cardiac, arterial and cholesterol problems; acid indigestion; cataracts; hyperactivity; concentration problems; and yeast overgrowth, resulting in *Candida albicans* and other forms of fungal infection, such as vaginal thrush.

## NATURAL FORMS OF SUGAR

Simple carbohydrates include sugars that occur as a natural part of food such as milk (lactose), fruit (fructose), grain (maltose), and glucose (found in the blood as a result of digestion). Glucose is the only source of energy that can be used by the brain. A low level of glucose in the blood will cut off supplies to the brain, resulting in feelings of anxiety and faintness, such as in low-blood sugar syndrome (hypoglycemia).

When a good nourishing meal is eaten and digested, there is plenty of glucose available to the brain and the body for energy. Any surplus is converted and stored away in the liver. The store lasts for twenty-four to forty-eight hours. Thereafter, additional glucose must be produced from the stores of fat in the body. This source of glucose comes in a "package." All the nutrients necessary for digestion and absorption are contained in the milk, the fruit or the grain. Therefore the body is not robbed. These are nutritionally superior foods, which nourish every cell in the body with protein, vitamins, carbohydrates, minerals and fats. (See the Body's Biological Eating Clock on page 75.)

Dr. Weston Price, a dentist who travelled extensively among people who lived on traditional diets, made some wonderful discoveries. His book *Nutrition and Physical Degeneration* shows the before-and-after effects of modernization. A simple life, lived in accordance with the natural seasons of the year, eating foods that grow within a certain radius, bestowed good health on the local community. Because of lack of transport, there was no sugar, white flour or canned food available. There was very little tooth decay. People were vital and healthy. As soon as processed foods became available, problems appeared. There was tooth decay, tuberculosis and difficulty in childbearing. The children were born with poor development of the jaw and the facial structure changed.

## OUR BONES, OUR BRAINS, OUR BEHAVIOR

Protein builds our muscles, bones and connective tissue. It participates in the production of digestive enzymes and of hormones such as insulin, and in the formation of antibodies in our immune system. Amino acids (the building blocks of protein, which the body can break down into the various parts) may be involved in the formation of chemicals vital for the brain functions that govern mood and behavior.

Proteins are one of the absolutely essential ingredients for living a healthy vital life. There is a minimum quantity we need to eat in order to remain healthy. This quantity depends on our growth rate, body size and the presence or absence of disease.

Our need for protein increases in infancy, during pregnancy and breastfeeding, in healing of the tissues following an accident, injury or operation, or when recovering from loss of weight. Our needs for complete protein increase at a "crisis" time; in general, we can recover very well with fish, white meat and a little red meat. Worldwide traditions of eating have always included such dishes as rice and beans, with added vegetables, herbs and spices, or lentils and barley as in soup, or couscous and chickpeas, whole-grain brown bread and baked beans.

## THE NEW FOUR FOOD GROUPS

Based on research in the United States, Japan, Germany, France, England and Ireland, foods are now grouped as follows:

1. *Whole grains.* Including whole-grain bread, whole-grain pasta (made from rice, millet and buckwheat), oats, barley, corn, millet, bulgar wheat, cereal grains, buckwheat, quinoa, spelt grain (the original wheat grain). These grains are rich in fiber, contain some protein, B vitamins and zinc.

2. *Vegetables, fruits and sea vegetables.* Excellent sources of body-cleansing fiber, vitamin C and other vitamins and minerals for whole-body health, beta carotene and antioxidants to protect the cells in the body from the ravaging effects of pollution, poor diet, stress and tension.

3. *Yogurt, cheese, cow's milk, sheep, goat or plant milk (soy milk, oat milk, rice milk, almond milk or nut milk).* Sources of essential fats and fat-soluble vitamins, some B vitamins and calcium, magnesium and phosphorus.

4. *Beans, peas, lentils, meat, fish, poultry, eggs.* Excellent sources of fiber from the legumes, also iron, B vitamins and minerals. The red meat is distinguished as the only source of valuable, easy to obtain vitamin $B_{12}$, which prevents pernicious anemia. Vitamin $B_{12}$ is essential for nerve health. It maintains the integrity of the myelin sheath of the spinal cord. Deficiency can cause symptoms such as mood disorders, mental slowness, memory defects. Smoking (because of the cyanide in tobacco smoke) may be implicated in eye problems, because it interferes with the absorption of $B_{12}$. According to research, this happens more in men who smoke than in women who do so.

Vegetarians are prime candidates for vitamin $B_{12}$ deficiency, because their diet is devoid of the most valuable sources — liver, kidney, muscle meat and some fish. Sea vegetables or plant sources must be relied on for this vitamin as part of a vegetarian diet. Fish sources include flounder, herring, mackerel and sardines. Supplementing the diet with a tonic that contains vitamin $B_{12}$ is one of the best ways to guard against this deficiency.

## Traditional Diets

In the late nineteenth century, Dr. Price studied the diet of the Scottish people. Native people of the Outer Hebrides ate oaten cakes, fish, eggs, oat porridge, some milk and butter. The Danish, Swiss and southern European people generally lived on black bread, fresh vegetables, fruit, meat infrequently and raw milk. The Peruvian people ate corn, beans, seeds, guinea pig meat, seafood, river plants and potatoes.

The early Greeks lived on barley-meal porridge, lentils, flaxseed, bread, greens, turnips and goat cheese. Meat was used at celebrations or in war-time only. Hippocrates lived to eighty-three years of age. He understood the needs of the human body instinctively and also through study. Today, we have scientific evidence pouring in to confirm his teachings.

Traditional diets across the world have the following in common:

- the diet is frugal
- the foods are whole food
- the foods are grown locally
- seasonal factors are observed — some foods are scarce at certain times of the year
- no chemicals are used
- cooking methods are slow

Such diets can be described as being low in calories, protein and fat, and high in complex carbohydrates.

## COMPLEX CARBOHYDRATES

Complex carbohydrates are found in grains, beans, seeds, nuts, vegetables and fruits. They are a perfect whole food, containing carbohydrate with some protein, fat, fiber, vitamins, minerals. The grain is revered in all cultures — it is associated with the rise of civilization all over the world. It comes closer than any other food from the vegetable kingdom to providing our bodies with all the building blocks, energy and fiber we need for our health. After the introduction of oats, rice, millet or corn to the diet, it takes only a few weeks for the complex carbohydrates to begin exhibiting their wonderful properties.

## THE BENEFITS OF COMPLEX CARBOHYDRATES

The fibrous parts of grains, beans, seeds, nuts, vegetables and fruits cause a change in the stools. In the West, stools tend to be small, hard and infrequent. This may be implicated in diverticular disease, irritable bowel syndrome or constipation, which afflicts so many people today. A diet combining whole grain beans, peas, seeds, nuts, vegetables and fruit produces a profound change in the colon and texture of the stool. A large, soft, easily propelled stool is the result.

The bran part of the complex carbohydrate (rice bran, oat bran, wheat bran, soy bran) has been recommended by many doctors for helping to maintain a healthy cholesterol level, thereby reducing strokes and heart problems. Because fiber is so low in calories and high in bulk, it produces a full feeling and prevents overeating. In addition, as the foodstuffs mentioned here provide the body with the B-complex vitamins and minerals, they support it in times of stress. They also provide the body with stamina, both mental and physical, because of the gentle, steady, slow release of sugar (glucose).

These foods need to be chewed very well in order to release the enzymes in the mouth that prepare them for easy digestion through the digestive tract. As they are chewed, they become sweet, satisfying and comforting.

## FAT IS ESSENTIAL FOR LIFE

The body needs fat, but also needs to receive fat in its most nutritious form. Saturated fat, which is contained in meat and dairy products, can cause high cholesterol; unsaturated fats need to be included in the diet as well. Unsaturated fats come in two forms. Most obviously, they are present in oils — for example, olive oil, sunflower oil, soy oil, butter, lard and cocoa butter. They are also an integral part of certain foods, especially whole grains, nuts, seeds and fish.

We depend on fat to deliver the fat-soluble vitamins A, D, E and K throughout the body. These vitamins carry out protective functions that prevent infections, skin lesions, poor circulation, night blindness and "dry eye." They are instrumental in the formation of strong teeth and healthy gums resistant to gum disease, and in the production and maintenance of healthy mucous membranes. All of them are helpful, along with the B-complex vitamins, for normal growth and development in babies, young children and teenagers. These vitamins are like busy mothers and fathers in the body — building, helping growth, protecting, forming new healthy cells, preventing severe bleeding and nourishing the cells.

## THE FRIENDLY ESSENTIAL FATS

We need to recall the most important function of fat in our food: it is a builder. Every cell in our body and brain has fat as the major component of the cell wall. Essential fats give our cells impermeable walls, which we need to keep out the viruses that surround us. By having regular meals composed of grains, vegetables and fish, we supply our cells with these vital substances. Medical science is discovering that these essential fats are an integral part of unprocessed, naturally grown, chemical-free foods.

## THE HEALING FATS

Fats have different functions in the body. The evening primrose plant, the beautiful borage herb and blackcurrants all provide GLA (gamma linoleic acid). Among the many functions it performs are improved circulation, reduction of inflammation and lowering of blood pressure in the arteries. It prevents cholesterol production, helps the T-lymphocytes in the immune system and enables us to burn fat instead of storing it.

Fish is a better source of these fats than meat. Evening primrose oil is recommended by doctors for skin problems, including dry skin, dandruff, dermatitis and eczema. Doctors acknowledge that the faulty metabolism of essential fats, or a deficiency due to a poor diet, is at the root of many of the problems they see daily in their practices. Many of the people who have suffered from psychiatric, behavioral, learning and menstrual problems, in addition to recurring viral or bacterial infections, have been restored to normal life by a prescription of the essential fatty acids both in the diet and in the form of evening primrose, borage or blackcurrant seed oils.

## HOW FAT SUPPORTS LIFE

Apart from the medicinal aspects of fat in our diet, fat has other roles to play. Fat adds warmth, comfort and taste to our cooking. It keeps us warm by raising our temperature in cold weather. Our body contours are provided by fat. Fat also acts as a vital reserve should our food supplies fail. Of the eight essential elements, our vitamin A and E come from the fat in our diet. When we eat a whole food diet, including a wide range of foods, these vitamins, the ordinary fats and the essential fats are all present.

## HOW TO ACHIEVE BALANCE

Replace refined sugar with fruit (including dried fruit), honey, maple syrup, raw cane sugar for cooking (in very reduced amounts), fruit purées and juices and carrot juice for baking. Replace heavy fatty foods with grilled low-fat foods, and replace red meat with vegetarian sausages and burgers. Introduce whole grain rice, millet, couscous or bulgar wheat instead of French fries. Fries are to be regarded as an occasional treat. Instead of buying ready-made soups and sauces, make your own.

The ideal diet contains approximately 25 percent fat, 15 percent protein and 60 percent carbohydrates. As you adjust your eating habits to obtain this balance, the new foods and extra water will act like brooms and brushes. Waste prod-

ucts that have been clogging up the cells for years will begin
to move out through the normal channels of excretion,
mainly the kidneys and the intestines. You may feel like you
are starving and unable to wait for your next meal. This is
because the body simply cannot get enough of the delicious,
nutritious food. This hunger does not last too long, though,
as you begin to efficiently digest, absorb and fuel the body
from the new diet in a few weeks. This is the food the brain
and body need — they love it!

About one quarter of our diet needs to contain fat. If we consider the foods that are natural bearers of healthy fats, we
are on our way. Sunflower, sesame and pumpkin seeds are
excellent sources. When shopping for oil, buy sunflower oil
— look for unrefined, cold-pressed varieties, in dark con-
tainers. Buy only small quantities and use very little in cooking. Use mainly as dressing on salads.

As your body adjusts to less fat, it also learns to utilize new
sources of proteins — less from processed foods, more from
fish, home-cooked vegetable and meat soups and stir-fry
foods. It is adapting to a greater variety of grains, brown
rice, millet, corn, which all supply some protein, a little fat
and plenty of carbohydrate. The protein we eat becomes the
building blocks of the brain and body.

### Health-Giving Fats

*The avocado* has lots of fiber and is a wonderful source of vitamins A, C, E and B complex, in addition to minerals and
potassium. Avocados as part of a healthy diet help keep our
circulation and heart supplied with excellent nutrition. Very
good for the skin, they help make collagen (which is under
our skin), and help maintain the elasticity and smooth,
wrinkle-free appearance of our largest body organ.

*Oily fish* such as sardines, mackerel and herring are re-
nowned as "brain food," helping brain function, eyesight

and learning ability, reducing cholesterol, thinning the blood and reducing the risk of blood clotting. Fish also helps balance the body's water levels.

*Nuts* such as almonds, hazelnuts, chestnuts, walnuts and Brazil nuts contain fats with life-giving enzymes, selenium, B complex, potassium, zinc, calcium, folic acid and iron. Only buy them from a source that has rapid turnover; otherwise, buy them in their shells.

## VITAMINS THAT FEED THE BRAIN

Our brain is the great broadcasting station upon which we depend. All our learning abilities, our creativity, our five senses, are the daily transmissions of this great organ. How do we keep ourselves oriented toward a positive, healthy brain with a good memory, good concentration and retention? How do we keep ourselves socially outgoing, feeling warm and caring toward our family and friends? The answer is simple — feed the brain.

Much has been said about the needs of the body. When we nourish the body with mineral- and vitamin-rich nutrition, certain organs, such as the liver, and the muscles become depots for the storage of energy. This is a miracle of economy by the body. The stored energy (called glycogen) can be called upon to help in a situation the body sees as an emergency — too long between meals, an injury, accident or emotional upheaval. However, if through lack of awareness or thought about the needs of our body we cause these to occur frequently, we will notice the effects. Easily fatigued or easily injured muscles, muscle cramps and restless legs are just some of the problems of depleted nutrition in the muscular body.

The brain has no such storage depots — it has no capacity to store energy. It needs to receive a constant supply of fuel from the blood. The heart pumps one quarter of its blood directly to the brain. If your meal has been poorly chosen — composed of white sugar, high fat, high salt, low fiber, few complex carbohydrates and essential fatty acids — the blood carries this nutrient-poor supply to the brain. Poor eating may be sufficient to deplete the brain of the constant supply of nourishing minerals, vitamins, enzymes, amino acids, glucose and oxygen necessary for it to do its work properly.

## FOODS THAT FEED THE BRAIN

Phosphorus-rich foods include the most well-known source: fish, also a rich source of iron, iodine, sulphur and zinc. Other important sources of phosphorus are almonds, protein drinks made from soy flour (available in health food stores), beans, cheese, wheat germ, wheat bran (from organically grown sources, so the bran does not have to compete for nutrients with pesticides), sunflower seeds, cashew nuts, Brazil nuts and whole soybeans (from an organically grown source only, to avoid genetically engineered foods).

## WINTER FOODS RICH IN IMMUNE-PROTECTING VITAMINS AND MINERALS

*Vitamin A (beta carotene)*   Yellow, deep orange and dark green vegetables and fruit.

*Vitamin B complex*   Almonds, whole grains, meat, poultry, cheese, fish, sunflower seeds, eggs, avocado, rice bran.

*Vitamin $B_{12}$*   Beef, beef liver (from free-range sources), eggs, flounder, herring, mackerel, milk, milk products, sardines.

*Vitamin $B_9$ (folic acid)*   Barley, calf's liver (free-range), beans, chickpeas, green leaf vegetables, lentils, whole grain rice, peas, split peas, sprouted seeds, wheat, wheat germ.

*Vitamin C*   Acerola cherries, blackcurrants, fruit, rosehips, broccoli, cabbage, parsley, potatoes, tomatoes, paprika, sprouts, lemons, watercress.

*Vitamin D*   Cod liver oil, salmon, sardines, tuna, butter, milk, eggs, cheese.

*Vitamin E*   All unprocessed seeds and nuts, whole unprocessed grains, green vegetables, evening primrose oil, borage oil, cold-pressed oils used as dressings in salads — soybean, safflower, wheat germ.

*Bioflavonoids*   Skin and pulp of fruits such as oranges, lemons, apricots and cherries, buckwheat, green peppers.

*Calcium*   Sesame seeds, tahini, hummus, fish, yogurt, cheese, milk, sea vegetables (carrageen, dulse, kombu, wakame), blackstrap molasses, kelp, tofu, leafy green vegetables, almonds, sunflower seeds.

*Iron*   Meat, egg yolk, sea vegetables, blackstrap molasses, chickpeas, lentils, mussels, pistachios, pumpkin seeds, walnuts, wheat germ.

*Magnesium*   Almonds, fish, leafy green vegetables, blackstrap molasses, nuts and seeds, soybeans, wheat germ. Many foods that are rich in calcium also have magnesium.

*Phosphorus*   Skimmed milk, wheat germ, soy flour, brown rice, whole-grain bread, almonds, dried beans, free-range calf's liver, cheese, eggs, fish, peas, poultry, seeds, sardines, tuna, whole grains.

*Silica*   Oats, soybeans, sesame, sunflower and pumpkin seeds, blackstrap molasses.

*Zinc*   All unprocessed whole grains, meat, poultry, fish, egg yolk, turkey, oysters, wheat germ, oat bran.

# 5

# CONSULTING A NUTRITIONAL THERAPIST

---

## Do I Need Nutritional Therapy?

How do you know whether you would benefit from nutritional therapy? The short answer is that everyone, whatever their state of health, is likely to benefit to some extent from looking carefully at their eating habits and making improvements as necessary. If you suddenly experience a change of health for the worse, such as the development of asthma, migraines or insomnia, your body is giving you clear messages that you need to reconsider both your eating habits and your lifestyle. On the other hand, many illnesses do not present themselves suddenly.

These are some indicators that your health is being undermined:

1. *Fatigue* Rest does not alleviate this form of tiredness. Even when you go to bed early and appear to sleep well, you wake up feeling tired.

2. *Irritability*   We are all irritable on occasion, but this is different. If you are chronically irritable, it means you become irritable for very little or no reason at all, probably due to a hormonal imbalance.

3. *Change of appetite*   Eating too little or eating too much can lead to great weight loss or gain.

4. *Energy loss*   If your energy is low, your immune system will be vulnerable, lowering your resistance to infection. You will be susceptible to regular colds and flu, especially in winter.

5. *Collapse*   Following a heart attack or irritable bowel syndrome, arthritis, diabetes, asthma or other illness that necessitates a visit to the hospital.

If any of these states describes you, it is advisable for you to seek the help of a professional nutritionist.

### FINDING A NUTRITIONAL THERAPIST

Once you have decided to consult a nutritional therapist, how do you set about finding one? The best way is probably by recommendation; seek advice from your local health-food store or library if you do not have friends who can put you in touch with someone they recommend.

### WILL VISITING A NUTRITIONIST AFFECT ANY MEDICATION I AM TAKING?

No. But if you are taking any medication, it is important that you give this information to your nutritionist. It will also help your nutritionist if you have recently had a complete physical, as this can narrow down the time it takes to identify the source of your problem. Nutritional therapy can work extremely effectively alongside orthodox medicine. If you have a medical check-up before visiting a nutritionist, you will probably find it interesting to have a follow-up visit a few months later, so that you and your doctor can establish the effects of your nutritionist's treatment.

## WHAT HAPPENS IN THE INITIAL SESSION?

When you meet your nutritional therapist for the first time, the consultation will probably last for an hour to an hour and a half. To gain a better understanding of your present needs, the therapist is likely to ask quite detailed questions about your personal history. You may be asked to describe your past as well as current lifestyle, including your eating patterns and your attitude toward yourself.

You may also be asked about your family's health history. This is because we all carry genetic weaknesses as well as strengths. It is true that within the same family each person is completely unique, with specific needs. At the same time, we all inherit tendencies we may be able to reverse once we become fully aware of them. Looking at your family history may show that you have inherited problems such as obesity, skin problems, constipation, poor circulation, chilblains or feeling the cold even in warm weather. Just because your ancestors suffered from these complaints does not mean you have to carry them with you through your own life.

### THE THREE CATEGORIES OF ASSESSMENT

The three categories of assessment I observe as a nutritional therapist are as follows:

1. *A thorough physical assessment*   A physical appraisal noting any current weaknesses or symptoms such as backache, headache, indigestion, breathing difficulties, etc., as well as a note of what form of exercise you do on a regular basis.

2. *An assessment of your family's health history*   This includes siblings, parents and grandparents; your personal health history from birth to the present, including recurrent patterns of illness or repeating symptoms, record of drugs, medication or vitamins used, including the periods of time over which they have been used.

3. *Dietary information*   Record what you ate as a young person growing up, which will give an indication of your ancestors' way of eating, as well as what you typically eat now.

4. *Blood, urine or hair analysis*   Your therapist may take samples and explain the results of the laboratory analysis at your next appointment.

## CREATING AN EATING REGIME

Together, you and your nutritionist will work out a revised eating regime, which may include mineral or vitamin supplements, depending on your state of health and lifestyle and on the nature of your specific problem. To do this, you will be asked to consider food in the widest sense, and to write out a brief account of what you are likely to eat over a period of a week. It is important that you do this as accurately as possible, because your account will reveal any strengths and weaknesses you may have both in the choices you make and in the way and the time you usually eat.

If your nutritionist suspects an allergy, you may wait until your second appointment to establish the results of a blood, urine or hair analysis, which will have identified the particular allergy. Depending on the extent to which your current eating habits are conducive to health, and on your condition, the changes in your diet may be significant and immediate or gradual. This is something you and your nutritionist are likely to work on together, but a typical change of shopping list will look like the following:

| Old Shopping List | New Shopping List |
| --- | --- |
| White bread | Whole-grain bread |
| Cereal | Sugar-free muesli |
| French loaves | Mixed seed loaves |
| Brown bread | Caraway seed rye bread |
| Black tea | Low-caffeine or herbal tea |

| | |
|---|---|
| Instant coffee | Fresh coffee |
| White sugar | Turbinado sugar |
| Sweet rolls and cakes | Whole-grain muffins |
| Cookies | Nuts and dried fruit |
| Chocolate | Carob |
| Meat | White fish |
| Fish in batter | Oil-rich fish (salmon, mackerel) |
| Chicken | Free-range chicken |
| Butter | Cold-pressed virgin oils |
| Whole milk | Nonfat milk |
| Canned vegetables | Fresh, organic vegetables |
| Fruit | Fruit in season only |
| Jam | Sugar-free fruit spreads |
| Ready-made desserts | Live yogurt |

## THE IMPORTANCE OF EATING REGULARLY

One of the keys to good nutrition is eating regular and balanced meals. Your nutritionist will probably encourage you to eat a good breakfast, a lunch that contains plenty of fresh vegetables and a light supper. If your caffeine intake is high, you will be advised to cut down on it and in some cases to eliminate it altogether. If you drink a lot of alcohol, you will be asked to reduce your intake.

Many simple problems, such as mood swings and low energy levels, are caused by a diet that is high in refined sugar and does not include a sufficient range of protein-rich foods. If this is your case you will probably be advised to include protein-rich drinks or snacks in your daily eating program, as well as a good breakfast, lunch and evening meal. Every person's eating requirements are unique, but for a typical, nutritious daily menu, see page 96.

## EXERCISE

If exercise is not part of your current lifestyle, your nutritionist will almost certainly recommend at least a twenty-minute walk each day. Regular exercise improves the metabolism and increases mental alertness. If you exercise well, you will start to digest your food more efficiently and sleep more deeply. Health, like illness, does not affect particular organs in isolation — it affects the whole person. Regular exercise plays an important part in maintaining a healthy lifestyle.

## AFFIRMATIONS

As you revise your eating habits and your attitude to life, you may find it helpful to use affirmations. Affirmations are a simple yet effective way of bringing about a long-term change of attitude and in helping banish old habits. They should focus on your present state; affirmations are not wishes! I find them most effective if they are repeated daily, on waking each morning and just before going to sleep in the evening. Typical affirmations about health are:

"I am expressing myself in positive ways."

"I feel light and buoyant and full of hope."

"I am becoming stronger and healthier every day."

## HOW MANY SESSIONS WILL I NEED?

The number of sessions will depend on the nature of your problem and on your ability to change your lifestyle in order to relieve the problem. It is impossible to say in advance how many sessions a person will need, because everyone is unique. Even if two people with similar lifestyles and family histories came to me with the same problem, I would not assume that they would both need the same treatment over the same period of time.

As the weeks progress, you will find that a great deal of nutritional therapy depends on your ability to help yourself. Your nutritionist is there to advise and guide you, but in the end you will be the one to make the changes.

6

# MONITORING PROGRESS

———

Changing old ingrained eating habits can be a challenging experience. To help keep up your morale and to monitor your progress as accurately as possible, it is recommended that you keep a daily food diary over a period of at least three months. Some changes in diet will have an immediate effect. Since the effects of certain foods are cumulative, however, benefits from these will occur at a deep level only with time. The changes your nutritionist recommends should not be seen as a short-term fix, but as the start of a change in your relationship to food that should last your lifetime. So keep in mind both the long-term and the short-term value of the food you are eating when you start your diary.

## KEEPING A FOOD DIARY

Use your food diary to record

- what you eat and drink, including quantity

- how you eat (with enthusiasm, resistance, enjoyment, quickly or slowly)
- the effects of what you eat — immediately after the meal and a few hours later

In addition to keeping this record, assessing your overall attitude to food after the first couple of weeks can be helpful. Your self-assessment may look something like this.

*LIFESTYLE AND FOOD*

| Old Thoughts | New Thoughts |
|---|---|
| Food was a means to an end, given little or no thought, as long as I had enough energy to get through my day | A new awareness of the importance of food in my motto "I need quality not quantity"; I want fresh food, which has higher amounts of the vitamins, minerals and enzymes needed to keep me healthy |
| Food was chosen for convenience, speed of preparation, minimum time spent cooking | I take pleasure in cooking with care and adding herbs to my meals |
| No association made between outbreaks of flu, colds, infections and the food being consumed | When I feel a cold coming on, I eat lots of fresh fruit and it goes away |
| Liquid intake meant copious cups of tea, occasional coffee or alcohol, fruit juices, high-caffeine drinks | Liquid intake means a glass of water at least three times a day; my new foods also provide a lot of liquid |
| Favorite foods were on my shopping list every day, including ones that were high in fat, sugar, salt, flavorings, additives, colorings, preservatives and, unknown to me, herbicides, pesticides, antibiotics, hormones and irradiation | I now look for "no artificial anything" on food labels — including sweeteners, sugar, salt, flavors, color or preservatives |

## Practicing Self-Observation

Look out for signs of deficiency in your diet. Do you look pale? Do you feel tired? Do you feel breathless after climbing up the stairs? If so, you need more folic acid, iron and foods rich in $B_{12}$. These include all kinds of greens and a little meat.

Because you are in a transitional phase in the first few months, your body is feeling the changes. Gradually, you will build up sufficient minerals, vitamins and essential fatty acids. These will strengthen not only your immune system but the trillions of cells that make you who you are — you will develop much greater resistance to colds and flu.

## Honoring the Digestive Process

Even a nutritionally rich meal can be undermined if it is not eaten in the right spirit. The following guidelines are basic to good digestion, and were once widely practiced:

1. *Quietness before starting to eat*   This was achieved in the past by having a quiet drink and a prayer before meals.

2. *Eating with enjoyment, awareness and gratitude*   In households where people love food, great discussion on the subject takes place.

3. *A half-hour period of rest or quiet after the meal*   Rushing back to work, brisk walking, heavy laboring work, playing any game in which there is strenuous physical activity and/or which involves keen concentration all interfere with the proper digestion and assimilation of food.

## Relaying Progress to your Nutritionist

Bring your food diary and any related notes to your appointments. Your nutritionist may be able to make connections that are not immediately apparent to you. He or she will also look at your overall health picture. Are you feeling less tired? Have you better, more steady energy during the day? Are your moods better? All of these questions are as important whether you are a man, woman or child.

Your diary will be of enormous help in reminding you how you were feeling six weeks ago compared with how you are now. Are you sleeping better, waking up refreshed? Although it may take three months to achieve correct balance throughout the hormonal system, good signs — such as less cravings for sugar, caffeine or nicotine, less bloating, less fluid retention — should become apparent after the first four to six weeks. Your body temperature should be stable and your circulation good. Your hair, nails and teeth should become stronger.

## ADJUSTING TO YOUR NEW EATING PROGRAM

Most people take quite a long time to feel comfortable with a new way of eating. After about six weeks, however, you should begin to feel quite relaxed with your program. You have now become expert at label reading. Shopping has a new function: to protect you from choosing incorrectly or unwisely. Recipes should be simply prepared, cooked according to your time available, and served quickly to enjoy all the benefits. You may be missing your sweet treats. You may need either to make your own or to try the delicatessen and health-food stores for homemade, high-fiber, low-sugar muffins, carrot cake, etc. Look for the yogurts containing *Lactobacillus bulgaricus*.

## THE SWISS NATURE DOCTOR

Dr. Alfred Vogel, the famous Swiss nature doctor, was born in 1902 and has been a practitioner since the 1930s. He has been responsible for much of the now widespread knowledge available on the subject of eating the "whole food way." His book *The Nature Doctor* has sold 2,000,000 copies, and has been published in many languages; it is the story of Vogel's life, detailing how he discovered the medicinal power of herbs, descriptions of how they work in the body and his herbal tincture formulations.

One of Dr. Vogel's many discoveries was made while working with clients in his clinic in Teufen in Appenzellerland. There he prepares extracts from fresh plants and uses them as medicine. He found that the tinctures made from the juice rather than the dried plant were more effective. Your nutritionist will choose from a wide variety of such herbal plants to help you. In the early stages of your eating-for-health program, it will be necessary to use these herbs and perhaps mineral and vitamin supplements to encourage the immune system to become strong.

## Sample Food Diary

### Day One, Week One

**Old Breakfast**
Refined cereal (low in fiber), white bread, jam, tea or coffee.

**New Breakfast**
Cereal (high in fiber, low in sugar), rice cakes with sunflower spread, sugar-free apricot jam, low-tannin, low-caffeine tea or coffee.

**11:00 a.m.**
Craving for something sweet or salty, also longing for tea or coffee.

**11:00 a.m.**
Have protein drink — feel quite nourished, have more energy, better concentration, better mood.

**1:30 p.m. Lunch**
Store-bought sandwich — cheese, egg, mayonnaise (high in fat) — and a canned soft drink (high in sugar).

**1:30 p.m. Lunch**
The protein drink's effects have lasted until now. This means I've made it through the morning since breakfast with minimal discomfort and the minimum of snacks and high-caffeine drinks. My healthier morning has helped me choose a healthier lunch, to eat slowly, enjoy and appreciate my meal. It was easier to choose yogurt instead of a rich

dessert. I enjoy meat, gravy for lunch and choose a yogurt for dessert.

**4:00 p.m.**
Feeling hungry. Would love a chocolate bar.

**4:00 p.m.**
Have protein drink and a high-fiber, high-protein bar to help me steer clear of the chocolate.

**5:00 p.m.**
On the way home from work — tired, hungry.

**5:00 p.m.**
Have bottled water in the car. Eat protein bar — feel better.

**6:30 p.m. Dinner**
Usually something fast, such as pizza or Chinese take-out or tacos. Fresh vegetables are reserved for weekends, when there is time to cook. Will make an effort to have a small amount of salad.

**6:30 p.m. Dinner**
Brought home quiche lorraine from the delicatessen, with two salads — broccoli with cashew nuts and pasta with celery, cucumbers, peas and corn. After dinner I allow myself a bag of chips as a treat. Feeling good.

## END OF WEEK ONE

I have had a reasonably good week. Made a good effort to keep to the program. Found the protein drink a life-saver! Could not have managed the discipline of keeping away from the refined sugars without it. The protein drink not only gave me a nice nourished feeling, but it seems to have reduced the severity of the withdrawal symptoms from sugar in general. I did have to have a bar of chocolate three times during the week, but I went to the local health-food store and bought a healthier alternative. I needed the chocolate when I ran out of supplies. Shopping is not easy when you are learning to read labels. A helpful hint — never go shopping when you are hungry! Do not bring either yourself or the children to the store until you have taken the edge off your appetite.

Day One, Week Two

*Breakfast*

I am loving my breakfast. This week I am having fresh seasonal fruit, with natural yogurt and a little fruit yogurt. I add sunflower seeds and hazelnuts for extra nourishment.

*11:00 a.m.*

I make my protein drink up with water and juice. I have my normal lunch, because it is familiar and comforting.

*4:00 p.m.*

This is definitely my low-energy time. The protein drink and bar are very helpful.

*6:30 p.m. Dinner*

A vegetable dish with breast of chicken is quick and tasty.

## End of Week Five

Have become quite an expert at label reading, so my "new" shopping is a lot easier. I have found some new substitute foods for old ones. There is a very good selection, for example, of muesli-type breakfast cereals. I have chosen a very basic one and add my own fresh fruit to it, with pumpkin seeds. There are many types of bread, including whole-grain bread, oat bread, rye bread and whole grain crispbreads with sesame seeds. Sometimes I have feta cheese, cottage cheese or vegetarian cheese instead of butter. My whole interest in food is changing — I am looking out for a much wider range than ever before. Consequently, my approach to my program has changed. This is an education in eating, not at all the narrow diet I thought would be my prescription.

Day One, Week Six

*Breakfast*

A glass of warm water. My nutritional counselor has now recommended this as a great way to start the day. Muesli, fruit, pumpkin seeds, granary bread, vegetarian cheese.

*11:00 a.m.*

Protein drink, crackers with sesame seeds (just in case!).

*1:30 p.m. Lunch*

I now choose extra vegetables to have with fish, chicken or meat. Most days a yogurt, occasionally fruit salad with cream.

*4:00 p.m.*

Protein drink. I keep my high-protein bar for the journey home, because it stops me from going into the store for a chocolate bar. I also have a handful of sunflower seeds.

*6:30 p.m. Dinner*

Lasagne with salad and whole-grain pasta.

## THE IMPORTANCE OF KEEPING A FOOD DIARY

Keeping a diary will enhance your sense of responsibility toward yourself; the combined knowledge of choosing healthier food and changing your eating habits will give you a feeling of being in control of your life. Gradually the cravings will disappear. You will start to appreciate your lunch and dinner more if they are thoughtfully prepared, well-balanced dishes rather than fast-food.

## RECOMMENDED FOODS

Chickpeas; homemade brown bread with added rice bran, oat bran or wheat germ; pancakes with added molasses (made from oat flakes, honey, sunflower oil, molasses with sunflower seeds and sesame seeds added); pumpkin seeds; almonds; parsley; watercress; sprouted alfalfa seeds; sprouted mung beans — small but very valuable sources of a whole range of vitamins, minerals and iron.

# 7

# NUTRITION AND
# THE ENVIRONMENT

When you feel quite well, having reached the stage where you are really enjoying your food, a new development takes place. Questions arise. What is in my food? How can I be assured of the quality of my food? How and where is it grown? You will want less food coloring, fewer preservatives. You will certainly not want food that has been chemically treated, genetically engineered, treated with hormones or irradiated.

Transporting and storing food had been a concern for every society since man stopped hunting and gathering. Both staples and luxury foods have always been processed for journeys beyond the stockade — or the grave. Every army has devised ways of carrying its rations and many of their techniques we still use today.

The Moghuls moved across Asia with flanks of salted meat strapped to their pack animals, and yak's milk in hides became cheese as the animals plodded along. The Plains Indians dried buffalo meat, which they secured in strips for when it was needed; this is still available as beef jerky, from when their technique was commercialized. Salted fish was taken on boats in the days before refrigeration, but it remains in the diet of seafarers even after they pull up anchor and become landlubbers.

More spectacularly, Napoleon Bonaparte took his cooks to war with him. That way they were on hand to honor his victories with new dishes such as "chicken Marengo" or "chicken Kiev." He knew his soldiers marched on their stomachs, and he employed good psychology.

## CHEMICAL FARMING

Chemical farming came into being with a great flourish around 1945, but was really being developed since 1918. With the use of mineral fertilizers rich in nitrogen, phosphorus and potassium, farming became a profitable business — agribusiness. Until then, agriculture had been mostly carried out on nature's terms. People had cooperated with the earth. The farming was based on the needs of the soil — the variety and rotation of crops, rest periods, and feeding the soil with compost or manure. Only a small number of traditional farmers remain at the end of the twentieth century. Their focus changed from feeding the locality to answering the needs of the food conglomerates.

The farmer of one hundred years ago knew by following the tradition of his forefathers that his methods were enriching, sustainable and safeguarding the future of the soil. Today, we have a farmer who produces technological food — and a confused consumer. It is time for consumers to ask the question: Where does responsibility for the safety of our food begin?

## PROFIT MARGINS

In a quest for even greater profit margins, scientists are ready to unleash their latest discoveries on the world: genetically changed plants and vegetables, programmed to grow and behave exactly the way scientists want them to.

The story of American breakfast food is that of the promotion of the Western diet. In the mid-1800s, a popular quick breakfast food was sold in small navy blue tubs, with the picture of a smiling Quaker on them; the connotations were of thrift, piety and colonic hygiene. Simple and regular. The Kellogg brothers then "invented" cornflakes; because they were soon in competition with each other, they had to invent ever more appealing packages.

Psychological appeal features from here on in the packaging and marketing. Eventually, the boxes became huge and brightly colored, with plastic "extras" inside and smiling Quakers replaced with *fun*. So our food comes to us now from the silo, wrapped in plastic, and we eat it on the run or whenever we want to enjoy ourselves. The early pioneers of these foods have become corporate America, which in turn is part of world conglomerates. They are now more involved in marketing and political lobbying than nourishing the nation.

Four multinational companies now control 87 percent of the world tobacco trade; three control 85 percent of the tea trade; three control 83 percent of the cocoa trade; three control 80 percent of the banana business; and five control 77 percent of the grain trade. Unlike governments, they are accountable to no one.

According to Paul Ross, in *World* magazine of November 1996:

> Today's unjust food trade system began in colonial times, when export or cash crops were given priority over subsistence crops that fed the local people. Profit margins have become the focus, and it will stay that way even though production is awry. We have mountains of food wasting away, or going to animal fodder, while people hunger everywhere. The old practice of subsidizing farmers to stop them

producing too much will probably be phased out soon as farmers give up their way of life.

Two new practices are being introduced by the mass producers of food, with only a cynical eye to the profit margin and no thought to the health of the public or the environment. Because of protests about preservatives in food, some producers now protect their crops by irradiating them. This practice is questioned by Dr. Earl Mindell:

> The purpose is to kill bacteria, fungi, insects and many undesirable creatures that may spread disease. The food does not become radioactive; however, irradiation does cause other changes in the molecular structure of food, notably an increase in free radicals (the unstable molecules that can cause other cells to mutate) and the formation of other potentially carcinogenic chemicals.

The other new threat looming on the horizon is food from genetically engineered crops.

## BRINGING IN THE HARVEST

The world's demand for corn was once met by the United States, but now China exports corn at the expense of its soybean crop. Meanwhile, the corn-depleted soil has been planted with soybeans as this is a leguminous plant that restores nitrogen to the ground.

The soybean, revered in Asia for centuries as "meat with no bones," was the first food to be engineered. In autumn 1996, they brought in the harvest in Missouri. The first genetically engineered crops were not openly identified as such — although they could have been, at the source — and once they came into the marketplace, they could not be distinguished from the normal crop.

*Talk Radio* in December 1996 posed the question, do we want this crop on our dinner table? The guest protesting against "gene-tinkering" was Dr. Richard Lacey of Leeds University, and he was supported by many of those who called in to the program. Dr. Lacey's argument was that this crop had not been tested. Surely, he argued, it was possible to do damage to growing organisms by feeding them material that had had its DNA manipulated to react to its normal environment in unpredictable ways. Going against the laws of nature meant nature might *not* heal anymore — where once meat was good, for example, it now meant BSE killed people. What would genetically-altered food do to us? We don't know. So let's find out *before* we all eat it unknowingly.

Greenpeace tried to stop the cargo boats, and the World Food summit in India was interrupted by protesters who claimed it could be a catastrophic mistake to allow genetically engineered food into our food chain.

## Consumer Choice

In Europe, 2,000 miles away, it looks as if consumers will not be given the choice. There will be no labeling to indicate the fact that the soybean is different. The engineered foods will only be a tiny percentage of the main crop, which is how they will be incorporated into the food chain. Foods that are expected to come into the marketplace soon are corn (insect-protected); canola (herbicide-tolerant); tomatoes and tomato paste (slow-ripening and non-squashy); sugar beet (herbicide-resistant); and cotton (bollworm-resistant). Others in the pipeline are chicory, tobacco, squash, canola, papaya, flax and brewer's yeast.

Research in Denmark has shown that genetically engineered resistance to an herbicide in oil-seed rape was transferred to weeds, which then passed it on to the next generation. Genetically engineered oil-seed rape is one of three crops that have been approved for Britain, the other two being the soybeans and corn. Already it has emerged that genetic engineering could result in crops that are harmful to health. When the Brazil nut was genetically transferred (i.e. through genetic engineering) to the soybean, it was quickly found to be allergenic — that is, anyone allergic to nuts was also allergic to the soybean. This project has since been abandoned.

## Silent Spring

*Silent Spring*, a classic study of the effects of pesticides, was published in the 1960s. Rachel Carson was the first woman to draw to the attention of the unsuspecting public the dangers of DDT. She named twenty-three other herbicides and pesticides as equally destructive to the life cycle of the soil, the creatures that lived on the plants from the soil, their reproductive cycle and the consequences for the new generation. Since then, hundreds of new chemicals have been introduced, and now among the public there is grave concern about the damage caused by them.

## What Is in My Food?

To answer this question, you need to know what *should* be in the soil. Good soil is crumbly in texture. In every inch of the soil there is a living microcosm by which the soil is both aerated and kept moisture-retentive. Tiny passages are created by the insects and earthworms that inhabit rich earth.

## The Tissue of the Soil

Fungal elements form a web that surrounds and penetrates the structure of plant roots, facilitating the plant's nourishment from the soil. Special soil organisms preserve the ability of the soil to survive variations in temperature, rainfall, frost and heat during each season. The soil provides nutrients for plants, which have water, carbon and nitrogen as their main constituents. The carbon material is the woody or fibrous part that, if not eaten by us or other animals, goes back into the soil and in some circumstances forms the peat or coal we burn. So we turn it into energy we call heat. If we eat this plant material, we turn it into the energy that is "being alive."

The nitrogen is held in the fibrous section, and reacts with the hydrogen and oxygen in our water and air, and with sunlight; it forms the green and leafy part of the plant. This, with the stems and roots, holds the vitamins, minerals and trace elements we need for our bodies to grow properly.

When we take a plant out of the soil, we remove material that we must replace if we want the same soil to keep producing for us. Simply to pump it with nitrate fertilizers is not to replenish it properly. This makes for unbalanced soil. We should put compost and manure back into the soil, and let the microorganisms and weather do the complex job of breaking down the nitrogen and carbon that is needed. Then we should plan our planting and harvesting around crop rotation.

## CROP ROTATION

Crop rotation is the three- or five-year planting plan a good farmer has for his fields. The same crop is not grown in successive years on the same plot; a waiting period of three to five years ensures that the soil has been "fed" and has absorbed the nutrients that were first removed with the harvest. In the in-between years, the farmer grows other crops that take a slightly different nutrient balance from the soil.

For example, a nitrogen-hungry plant like sweet corn is grown one year, with soybeans grown the next year. The beans, like all legumes, have nodules on their roots that store nitrogen the rest of the plant has drawn in. So when the soybeans are harvested, the root is left in the ground; as it breaks down and decays, it leaves a little more nitrogen behind than other plants would — especially the corn plant.

If the farmer planted squash after the soybeans, he would be taking very little nitrogen from the soil, because squashes are mostly water. This is a pattern of planting perfected by the Indians of Central America a thousand years ago. They not only fed themselves well without chemical fertilizers, but also invented our most famous breakfast food — the cornflake.

The rotation of crops practiced by most farmers before the end of the Second World War conserved the fertility of the soil. Tended with smaller machinery and shallow digging tools, the soil increased in depth and fertility almost indefinitely. The top soil became nutrient-rich, and it resisted the climatic tendency to wear it away.

### DAMAGE TO THE STRUCTURE OF THE SOIL

Once the application of fertilizer began, there came a great demand on the soil for increased production. Crop yields have increased, soil richness has decreased and the tissue containing the microorganisms has been damaged. Worms and insects are fewer in number; the soil structure has begun to degenerate. The production of high-yielding crops has resulted in stripping the fertility needed for the next generation.

### THE DISAPPEARING TOPSOIL

We have lost at least 250 billion tons of topsoil into the oceans. This lost topsoil has taken with it the nutrients necessary to maintain the life cycle of the soil.

In the thirty years since Rachel Carson sounded the alarm, there has been a thirty-fold increase in the use of pesticides. The new products may break down more quickly but they are equally toxic.

The Pesticide Action Network (PAN) has been campaigning for years for the prohibition of the "Dirty Dozen," including three chemicals identified by Carson and still in use today. The Pesticide Exposure Group of Sufferers has estimated that 2,500 of its 6,000 members have been damaged by organophosphates (OPs), which were developed from nerve gases. They are used mainly in sheep-dipping. Symptoms of mild OP poisoning are flu symptoms, headaches, fatigue, dizziness; acute poisoning can be fatal.

## QUALITY CONTROL

How can you be assured of the quality of your food? You may be lucky enough to have access to a retail outlet that displays a great deal of information about your food. Clear signs inform you of the farm from which the meat came, how the animals were fed (on grass or feed), the age at which the animals were slaughtered. Of great concern now to the consumer is the manner in which the animals have been reared, whether they have been humanely handled throughout their lives. There is an obvious difference between well-treated animals and those that are just a business investment.

## FRUITS, VEGETABLES, HERBS AND SPICES

Similar signs are necessary to indicate where vegetables and fruits originate from. Choices available to you should be

- no artificial fertilizer residue
- no toxic chemicals used after harvesting
- no cosmetic wax coating
- no artificial coloring
- no irradiation
- no genetic or transgenic engineering
- herbs and spices as nature intended — *natural*

## *HOW TO USE YOUR POWER AS A CONSUMER*

Constant dialogue with your producer, supermarket manager or local farmer creates a greater awareness of your needs as a consumer. The more people insist on having organic produce in their local stores, the more likely it is that the trends of intensive chemical farming will be reversed. This will safeguard not only your own health but that of future generations. The soil will then be fertile for generations to come, the cycle of wildlife will have established a flourishing habitat and the birds will have returned. The life of the earth will be secured.

RECYCLING, COMPOSTING — AND WHY

In the hot weather of July 1994, I was visiting a friend in the Midlands of England. I arrived with a large box of nectarines I had bought locally — there was a glut, and they were very inexpensive. They were not grown in Britain, but were a European product, and they tasted wonderful. My friend told me her pregnant daughter was having cravings for this fruit and liked to eat five or six a day. They both decided that it was all right to do so, as this was fresh fruit. What could be wrong with that?

On the second evening of my visit, we listened with horror to the evening news: there was a warning that adults should not eat more than two of these nectarines per day, and children one every other day, because many people were having allergic reactions to them. It was presumed the fruit had been treated with something toxic. In near panic my friend phoned her daughter — she could only think of the worst possible scenario for her unborn grandchild.

Alan Gear wrote in the *Henry Doubleday Research Association (HDRA) Newsletter* in 1993:

> Although there is a great deal of public unease over the use of pesticides, few people have first-hand experience of acute poisoning by these chemicals. The fear is based on the possible harmful effects of accumulating pesticide residues over many years of eating conventional food and drinking water contaminated with pesticides. Such compounds are known to cause cancer and genetic damage at high doses in laboratory animals. How can we be certain they are safe at current levels?

> The World Health Organization estimates that every year 3 million suffer acute, severe pesticide poisoning, of which over 20,000 may die. Much of this human tragedy takes place in developing countries where, worldwide, around 25 million people are

thought to be adversely affected by sprays one way or another.

Gear had just returned from Venezuela and gave a short review of the effects of the downturn in the country's fortunes since the decline in the oil market. As a result of economic need, farmers were encouraged to concentrate on intensive fruit farming. This necessitated big expenditures in chemical treatments to maximize yields. However, the farmers could no longer tolerate the expense involved — both to their finances and to their health.

> But it was what they had to say about pesticides that really caught my attention. One farmer reported that over forty people in his village had been poisoned by eating contaminated food. A speaker from Brazil showed a distressing set of slides of babies born to wives of agricultural workers. All had serious birth defects like extra or deformed limbs, or absence of eyes. Of eighty or so Andean farmers in the audience, none used any protective clothing or took any precautions when spraying. Pesticides were frequently broken down into unlabeled containers. Instructions, even when they could be read, were rarely followed. Many of the chemicals were banned in the West. Is it surprising that human health suffers?

> While I was out of the UK, the *Observer* newspaper ran a story alleging a possible link between the fungicidal benomyl, better known to gardeners as Benlate, and clusters of children in Lincolnshire born without eyes. Apparently in a Californian study, 63.5 percent of pregnant rats dosed with high levels of benomyl and fed on protein-deficient diets developed severe ocular anomalies.

The seasonal applications of these poisons are not the only source we have to worry about: we must remember they are recycled with crop residues and build up in the soil. The soil could be thought of as the earth's placenta — primitive people would have a clear idea of this as a part of Mother Earth, but for us "Mother" as a name for the earth has become a cliché. Yet the earth's soil, water and atmosphere nourish us and recycle our waste so we can feed again. We all know what happens to the embryo or child when a mother is sick.

Where there is no topsoil, there is no support system for higher life forms. An inch-thick layer — 150 metric tons of soil over a hectare — would take hundreds of years to develop without human or animal intervention. But when we and animals intervene to generate and exploit topsoil, we can produce massive layers in a relatively short time. This is not always the clean soil we need, however, and we must acknowledge its use to us and our responsibility to it.

One approach to cleaning up the soil and water and keeping ourselves healthy is to recycle organic matter and avoid the use of poisons. Even if you are not fortunate enough to live in a community that promotes diligent sorting and recycling, the composting of organic wastes to promote healthy soil and clean food can be easily managed on an individual basis. So let's make compost part of the earth's maintenance diet.

## COMPOSTING

Compost bins are vegetarians, although many minute and not so small life forms live in them. The first stage of decomposition of organic waste takes place by the interaction of air, water, microbes and heat. This starts the breakdown of nitrogen and carbon materials to make humus, which then becomes food for large and small organisms in the compost heap. So long as there is humus, there are organisms feeding off it and making plant nutrients. Even when the compost has been spread as a soil additive, microorganisms remain in it, keeping it healthy; after we have harvested the crop, they remain ready to take in more compost with which the depleted soil should be renewed.

Some of the most easily recognized inhabitants of the compost heap are the reddish and lumpy earthworms. They are not found in garden topsoil, for they work directly on the soft vegetable matter. And for this to happen the vegetable scraps must be collected in a warm, moist environment, like the center of a compost heap. Then vast numbers of earthworms come up from somewhere deep in the ground. Alone in a bin with kitchen waste, kept in a warm place, they will make a rich soil that is more a fertilizer than a growing medium. In the compost heap, where there is also woody, fibrous material to be broken down, the end product has a different composition and is the result of a complicated team effort. It is the dark, odorless, friable tilth we call "gardeners' gold," or compost — Mother Earth's favorite meal.

The results of many trials are available to show the greater capacity of composted soil to germinate seeds as compared with untreated soil; they also show how plants raised on composted soil give greater yields and are more disease-resistant.

These trial results illustrate that not only is it wasteful of resources — it is in fact criminal to continue applying artificial fertilizers and pesticides when plants thrive, untreated, in composted soil. Healthy soil is host to the predators of crop pests, and the vigorous plants that grow in composted soil are less prone to disease. When poisons are no longer applied to crops, the earth will start to heal — and so, therefore, will we.

## SIX SORTS OF COMPOSTING

**Field-sheet composting**   This is a farmers' technique. The residue of a food crop, such as sweet corn or cabbage, is left on the soil surface after the crop has been harvested. It breaks down partially by exposure to weather and is then plowed into the topsoil.

*Silage*  Another farming technique. A crop of "green manure" is harvested while sappy and fresh, and buried or tightly wrapped. The material is subject to a non-aerobic composting.

*Field windrows*  A farmers' or park-keepers' technique. The wastes from harvesting or pruning are stacked up in heaps or rows and periodically turned or added to. Roughly-hacked coarse material is used, so the result is a coarse humus that is best laid on the topsoil to protect it during winter rains. It is also very effective when laid around the base of plants that are subject to suffering during drought. In both cases, the composted material stays on the surface and is not worked in. It is integrated into the topsoil very slowly, which is why it is a useful shield.

*Compost heap or bin*  A gardeners' technique. Hacked autumn and spring prunings are mixed with soft sappy material, such as kitchen vegetable waste and discarded garden plants. The heap is added to at irregular intervals, and varying quantities of materials are added to top it off.

*Compost tumbler or tub*  Also a gardeners' technique. This is similar to the compost heap, but on a smaller scale, and the hacked material is contained in an enclosed bin that is either rotated or has the contents stirred at regular intervals. Because the smaller volume of material does not generate any heat, the decomposition process must be aided by insulation and human intervention.

*Worm bin*  The non-gardeners' technique. A container with a lid houses the earthworms on a layer of coarse sand, and they are fed with kitchen vegetable wastes. These then turn into a rich fertilizer/compost that is scooped out of the bin. Because the worms don't like frost, the bin should be kept in a shed, cellar or stairwell. The yield is small, but its quality compensates for the lack of quantity. It makes a great fertilizer for house plants.

Kitchen and garden wastes not processed by the household are collected in Bio-Bins by conscientious communities, but if these are not available, give the wastes to a friend or neighbor who composts — there's always a shortage of material.

## WHAT GOES INTO THE COMPOST BIN?

Any clean vegetable matter, but not roadside plants, because these may be contaminated with heavy metals from motor exhausts. The only animal products that can be processed are feathers and manure. Products such as blood, fishmeal and bonemeal are well-known fertilizers; these are usually worked into the topsoil in very small quantities, even if the soil contains compost. Paper in small quantities is all right as long as it has no printing ink on it (the ink contains toxins). Cooked vegetable material can be included, but avoid any mixed with dairy products. These are almost always oily, and oils block the ventilation of the mass.

Some large fruit seeds like those from mangoes or avocados take years to break down. So do nuts in their shells. Both can start sprouting in the soil long after they have been applied to the compost. All compost material should be seed-free. Try to remove all ripe seed heads; if this is not possible, don't include the plant. All material should be disease-free, and if firm and woody, it should be chopped. A chipper is a good investment. They aren't cheap, but you may be able to work as a cooperative, sharing the cost with a group. Material that is very wet will not go through the chipper, but wet materials can be put directly into the compost heap (which should always be kept moist).

Special additives, such as seaweed and wood ash, are very beneficial in small quantities. Very large quantities of grass-cuttings should be separated into small batches. While they are a good material, to dump them in straight from the mower could stifle the mass when they start to "mush," which happens very quickly. Yarrow, comfrey and nettles, on the other hand, can be added in batches — the bigger the better.

Evergreens, even finely chipped, don't break down well; conifers also contain a pungent resin that is not beneficial to the compost mass. Autumn leaves gathered into large heaps are best left to rot down on their own, and make a marvellous humus called leaf mold. Despite its name, it is not moldy; on the contrary, it's another form of "gardeners' gold." But if only small amounts are available, they go into the compost bin.

## WHAT DOES COMPOST HAVE TO DO WITH RECYCLING?

Site your compost bin or pile where you don't have to look at it all the time, but where you can still reach it easily. You will be gathering up all vegetable wastes and trimmings and collecting to keep the pile fed. The whole environment will improve before you have even applied any compost to the soil. The compost bin is just a cage or retaining wall for a compost pile; neither has a base, because the earthworms must come up into the pile from the ground when the pile first appears; then they disperse once the soft material is processed. The proportion should be twenty-five or thirty times more woody, fibrous matter than green, soft material. This breaks down to 15:1 carbon to nitrogen in the final product, which is considered the ideal ratio. To achieve a good rate of decomposition, the volume of material is important; it is best to gather unmixed materials in some bulk before layering them in a pile. In two or three days, the volume will have reduced dramatically, and if you pull the unchanged materials from the sides into the middle, this will generate another heating up period.

Your pile should have started with a mass of at least 1.5 cubic yards. Less volume than this will not heat up. Obviously, warmer weather helps the process, and in colder regions it is advisable to have solid walls for the bin but still allow air into the mass by turning it regularly. Keep heavy rainfall out of the pile. The material is ready to be applied to the topsoil when it has become the texture of soil; if some rough bits remain, sieve them out or leave them in depending on your gardening needs.

## WHY GO TO SUCH TROUBLE?

Because the alternative is killing us. Yes, for composting you need material, space, time and patience. And for the community collections you need good civic organization. But the material is free, and if we clean up a bit, the space is there. Only time is short. Too many of us are already suffering with everything from allergies to cancer; the news is nearly always resonant with the latest environmentally related health scare, which is the result of too little awareness of the organic world. We should stop *thinking* about it and *demand* organically grown food. With solidarity, we could — like a compost heap — become a critical mass; then we could use the energy it takes to attend to our ailments and illnesses to generate change. We must all recognize that we have been sick long enough, and that much of this sickness is a result of what we've done to Mother Earth.

# 8

# NUTRITIONAL THERAPY AS PREVENTATIVE MEDICINE

---

## MONICA

Fourteen years ago, a decision was made that would have repercussions for everyone throughout the world. It was the beginning of a study called MONICA (Multinational Monitoring of Trends and Determinants in Cardiovascular Disease), which was undertaken by the World Health Organization. It was the most ambitious study on the health of people's hearts and circulatory systems. It encompassed the continents, from Australia through Europe. The cost was an enormous $32 million, and more than ten million men and women were involved in thirty-nine population centers.

### HEART DISEASE IN THE NORTH AND SOUTH

As the results became available, a clear pattern emerged: the further north you live, the more likely you are to die of a heart attack. Take two cities — Belfast in Northern Ireland and Toulouse in southern France. The heart disease rate per 100,000 people in Belfast (in the age group forty-five to fifty-four) is 237; in Toulouse, it is 56 per 100,000. In the age group fifty-five to sixty-four, the contrast is even greater — 761 per 100,000 in Belfast, 175 in Toulouse.

Why is there such a remarkable contrast between living in the north and the south? Why should people living in the industrially developed north, with all its wealth, suffer such a high rate of death from heart and vascular disease? What are the protective factors, obviously missing from the northern climes, that are to be found in the south? These questions became even more puzzling, because MONICA studies showed no significant differences in cholesterol, blood pressure or smoking (the three classic indications for heart disease developing) in the countries studied. The deeper the investigations progress, however, the more clearly we see our answers. Part of the modern world has forgotten the culture of traditional eating. It is clear that southern Europeans know something about diet that northern peoples have forgotten — or, at least, are no longer practicing.

## THE EXAMPLE OF FRANCE

For thirty years, Dr. Serge Renaud, the French epidemiologist and director of Nutritional Studies at France's National Institute of Health and Medical Research, had been studying the effects of food on people in France. The MONICA figures showed that heart disease was highest in countries such as Ireland and Scotland on the one hand, and Australia and the U.S. on the other, while France was at the bottom. France was surpassed only by the Japanese traditional diet of rice, eaten with fish, vegetables, sea vegetables and meat.

The French have a similar blood pressure and cholesterol count as people in the U.S., but they outlive Americans by four years or more, suffer less than half the number of heart attacks, and yet smoke and drink more. This became known as the "French Paradox." Dr. Renaud was called out of the anonymity of his work to shed light on the puzzle. This he did through a five-year study, completed in 1993, which proved to be a showpiece for the influence of food and eating patterns on health.

Renaud demonstrated his research by taking 600 people who already had cardiac problems and were on a medically recommended diet for heart attacks. He put 300 of these on his own dietary program; the other 300 remained on their own diet. After five years, the results of the study showed a 76 percent decrease in the chances of a second heart attack for those following Renaud's dietary guidelines. This confirmed the results of his thirty years of work in the field, and the MONICA report.

In addition, it coincided with and confirmed the results of the EPIC report (European Prospective Investigation into Cancer and Nutrition), also published in 1993. The population of the northern countries is at greater risk of getting cancer than that of the southern countries. Luxembourg and Belgium lead the mortality figures for men, Denmark and the UK for women. Greece, Portugal and Spain are at the bottom.

## DIFFERENCES IN DIET

The helpful foods are as follows: vegetables — fresh, dried or frozen; grains — including bread, pasta, wheat germ, whole brown rice, couscous, bulgar wheat; fruit; low-fat vegetarian cheeses; yogurt; cottage cheese; small amounts of oil, olive oil (cold-pressed, virgin); small amounts of low-fat spread; fish; and white meat.

By contrast, foods likely to be detrimental to health are fatty and processed meat; meat preserved with nitrate salt and sugar; factory-farmed meat; factory-farmed chicken; factory-farmed eggs; hard fats — lard, suet, meat drippings; and full-fat cream, cheese and yogurt (especially when pasteurized and processed with other additives).

In 1993, a major international conference on the subject of nutrition and public health called Diets of the Mediterranean was held in Cambridge, Massachusetts. It was remarkable for at least two reasons. Present at the conference was Ancel Keyes, aged eighty-eight, a man in robust good health whose message of forty years previously had been rejected. A great pioneer of modern nutrition, Keyes was the first person to demonstrate the relationship between food intake and heart disease.

In his study, which took place in Naples in the 1950s, Keyes had observed that the wealthy population ate more butter, milk and red meat, and that they had much higher rates of death from heart disease than the less well-off. The Neapolitan people made great use of vegetables, fruit, pasta and bread. They ate little meat, used olive oil instead of butter and drank wine rather than milk.

Keyes carried out further research in Greece, where he became convinced that the healthiest diet resembled what the people of the Mediterranean had been eating for thousands of years. His intuitive correlation of information has now been scientifically confirmed. A high-fiber diet, with plenty of vitamins, minerals, enzymes, essential fats, natural sugars — and moderation — offers protection against disease of the circulatory system.

Only four years ago, Dr. Martijn Katan, director of the Department of Human Nutrition at Wageningen University in Holland, made another brilliant discovery. Hard margarines — accepted for years as a healthy substitute for butter — were just as unhealthy, but for an entirely different reason. Katan discovered that hydrogenation, the process that converts liquid vegetable oil to solid or semi-solid spreads, creates trans-fatty acids, which raise the level of LDLs (low-density lipids — regarded as bad cholesterol), and leads to clogging of the arteries.

The results of EPIC are now being fully explored. According to Dr. Elis Riboli, head of the nutrition and cancer program at the International Agency for Research on Cancer, we are now seeing that what puts you at risk for cardiovascular disease puts you at risk for cancer. A diet that's rich in fresh fruit and vegetables reduces the risk of most forms of cancer by 50 percent or more.

## CLASSIC DIETS OF THE WORLD

### *MEXICAN/MEDITERRANEAN/BALKAN*

#### THE SOLANACEAE FAMILY
Tomatoes and eggplants

#### THE CAPSICUM FAMILY
All peppers

#### THE CUCURBITACEAE FAMILY
Zucchini and all squashes

Mediterranean cuisine is rich in grains, legumes, fresh fruits and vegetables. Grain and legumes are a terrific source of fiber, which may protect against colon cancer. Fresh fruit and vegetables are loaded with fiber, as well as beta carotene, vitamin C and other important plant chemicals that may protect against heart disease and cancer.

The Mediterranean diet is short on processed foods, which may be packed with preservatives and saturated fat, and stripped of fiber and nutrients. Meat that is loaded with fat is used sparingly. Eggplant, tomato, pepper, garlic and onions are dietary staples; these are all foods that are currently being investigated by the National Cancer Institute for potential cancer-fighting properties.

The Mediterranean diet also calls for an abundance of herbs and spices, such as rosemary, sage, thyme and cumin. Many of these herbs and spices are potent antioxidants, which may protect against atherosclerosis by preventing the oxidation of LDL cholesterol, which is believed to be a major factor in the formation of plaque (plaque deposits on the arterial wall prevent the flow of blood to vital organs, including the heart).

In many Mediterranean countries, dinner is washed down with a glass of red wine. Red wine contains resveratol, a substance that appears to lower cholesterol. For further information, see *Food as Medicine*, by Earl Mindell (Fireside, 1998).

### THE JAPANESE AND MARITIME DIET

These diets have the highest intake of marine or Omega 6 fatty acids. These are even better than the terrestrial-based Omega 3 fatty acids in nuts and seeds. Also eaten in abundance are mushrooms and algae (seaweed); green tea is consumed.

### THE CHINESE AND KOREAN DIET

In this diet, many stock-based dishes, containing mostly liquid with rice and a little meat (which has been de-fatted by being boiled), are typical. Also eaten are fresh sprouts. The stocks themselves are infusions of herbal roots: ginger, galangal, lemon grass, ginseng and licorice. As in Japan, green tea is consumed.

See Appendix One for further information on herbs, vitamins, minerals and the properties of foods.

# 9

# CASE STUDIES

────

## CASE ONE: MARY

Mary is a twenty-five-year-old woman. She has eaten a very poor diet since she was a teenager — and "always got away with it," she says. Since Christmas she has had spells of extreme pain, shooting from underneath her front lower rib down through her hip, through to the right of her back and up into the middle of her back. This pain is always accompanied by nausea, weakness, complete loss of appetite, and thirst. Following tests, her doctor diagnosed a gallstone.

*DIET*

Mary eats nothing for breakfast and does not drink any water. At 10:00 a.m., for her work break, she has strong coffee with milk and a few cookies. For lunch at 1:00 p.m., she has French fries, a bar of chocolate and coffee. During her 4:00 p.m. work break, Mary has more strong coffee and cookies.

At dinner time she eats take-out pizza or Chinese food; later in the evening she has coffee and potato chips.

This "diet" consisted of very little besides fat and caffeine. There is no fiber worth mentioning, no liquids, no vegetables, no fruit, no grains, virtually no protein and plenty of salt and sugar, although they are hidden in the fast foods and cookies.

### General State of Health

Mary does not exercise because she's chronically tired. Her back was in continuous pain. Her breathing capacity was very poor due to smoking. The personal history questionnaire she filled in showed a digestive system problem and a very poorly functioning bowel — due in part to the poor diet, and to the sluggish state of her liver and gallbladder.

### Observations

A very interesting correlation between the times of the bouts of severest pain and Mary's diet was confirmed by looking at the calendar: Christmas, New Year, Easter, holidays and birthdays. Mary readily admitted to consuming more coffee, more refined foods and alcohol on all of these occasions.

### Treatment Program

Because Mary had come along at the request of her concerned boyfriend — who is very health-conscious and recognizes that Mary has an addiction to caffeine — I asked her permission to set out a nutrition program. Would she feel ready to take full responsibility for her own health? Would she be prepared to make more effort to apply the principles of the "four doctors":

- sun/air
- exercise/rest
- good food
- good water

Mary's answer was: "I am prepared to do anything necessary."

I drew three charts for her, which were to go up on the refrigerator door. Every day, Mary is to remind herself about the stress-sugar cycle and the body clock for eating times. When she learns to stay within the framework of both, she will regain control over her life. The three charts became Mary's guidelines.

My nutritional advice to Mary was as follows:

Begin the day with a large glass of warm water. Take one teaspoon of olive oil (virgin olive oil, first pressing) to help the digestion. For breakfast, have an apple, pear, peach *or* a handful of grapes; a slice of whole-grain bread, with sugar-free jam *or* marmalade; and a cup of chamomile or peppermint tea. Both these teas are good digestive aids, calming, soothing, allowing the digestive system to work in such a way that the person feels lighter and brighter. A cup of light

*THE BODY'S BIOLOGICAL EATING CLOCK*

*Elimination Phase*
4:00 a.m.–1:00 p.m.
The body
eliminates all
the waste
from the
previous
cycles.

*Digestive Phase*
1:00 p.m–8:00 p.m.
The body
has greater
digestive
power.

*Assimilation Phase*
1:00 a.m.–4:00 a.m.
The body has a full-time job
of assimilation of food.

*LOW BLOOD SUGAR CLOCK*

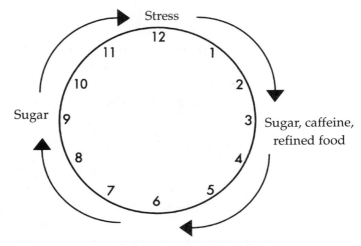

The results are mood swings from high to low,
anxiety, depression, poor energy levels

*LOW BLOOD SUGAR CORRECTION CLOCK*

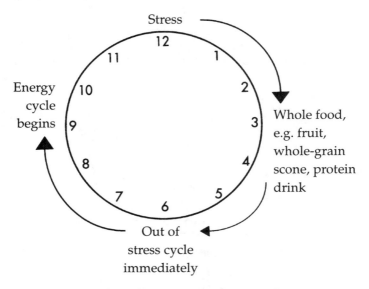

There is an even release of energy for hours,
mood normal, with a sense of well-being

tea *or* grain beverage at work. If she felt the need for a cup of real coffee, she was to make it weaker than usual. Lunch was to be brown bread *or* scone; fish *or* chicken *or* turkey; natural yogurt; and fresh fruit. Dinner gave Mary quite a lot of scope: vegetables in great variety, with rice *or* pasta *or* potato; fish *or* vegetarian tofu, *or* risotto, *or* vegetable and rice stir-fry, *or* vegetable lasagne, *or* shell pasta with tuna, onion, parsley and a little good-quality oil. (All pasta, rice and grains to be whole-grain.)

Mary has decided to wean herself off coffee over a six-to eight-week time span, by slow reduction, and by introducing a range of simple herbal teas.

## SHORT-TERM OUTCOME

After one month on this program — greatly helped by her boyfriend and her mother — Mary had a list of small but significant improvements. Her pain had eased within one week. In fact, she observed that after eating her meals according to the plan, she experienced freedom from acid indigestion, belching and bad breath. She was aware of her improved hair and skin — which had been blotchy, with angry red patches at times — due to all the good food and plenty of water. Mary's energy levels were slightly better; while she missed the caffeine, Mary realized she was on a much more even keel mood-wise than previously. She now had regular bowel movements instead of her previous irregular pattern (perhaps only once every three days).

Mary is enjoying the new wide way of looking at food, with better variety in all her meals. Looking at her charts helped her make out a shopping list, and she also avoided shopping when feeling very hungry.

## RETURN VISIT

Kinesiology testing on this visit suggested that her stone was now more gravelly; in fact, it seemed to be dissolving.

This was due to the effect of the pectin in the fruits, the olive oil in her diet (taken on a daily basis), all the vitamin-A rich vegetables, the plentiful supply of water, brown bread and the herbal teas. Kinesiology is a system of biofeedback from the body, using muscle testing. It is based on the principle that certain muscle groups are related to specific parts of the body. Such tests are used to detect and rectify energy blockages and any imbalances that cause illness. The practitioner uses light touch and deep massage, and gives dietary advice.

A big bonus was that her back now felt much stronger, due to the mineral-rich foods being absorbed into the bloodstream.

The only supplement added to her program was organic aloe vera, to encourage gentle improvements in the entire digestive system. Her eating program remains the same, although she is encouraged to shop for wider varieties of all types of foods on her menu. Special foods for Mary included the following: apples, apple juice, artichokes, beets, beet juice, carrots, carrot juice, cranberries, sugar-free cranberry juice, dandelion instead of lettuce, dandelion tea *or* coffee, garlic, grapefruit (pink), olives (unsalted), parsley, parsley tea, pears, red radish, white radish (mooli), water (pure).

## LONG-TERM OUTCOME

What began as a gallstone for Mary became at the end of her treatment program a small amount of broken stone (gravel), which the body can further break down and discharge slowly. This resulted from the nutrients and diet Mary was on. This is the process of cleaning the liver and gallbladder naturally. Follow-up treatment will continue to use very gentle effective herbal tonics to maintain Mary's general health and continue the process of breaking down the stone. In all cases such as Mary's, we ask the patient's doctor to monitor his or her progress.

Under the supervision of her doctor, Mary has continued to become healthier, with a renewed interest in her own ability to have beautiful skin, hair, nails, teeth and bones. She has a healthy appetite, good energy and is pain-free — all her systems are "go."

## Case Two: Jean

Jean remembered being a hyperactive twelve-year-old. The diet which was recommended for her did not help, and she had been off dairy products at the time; there was no beneficial result. She has recently married.

### Diet

Jean and her husband Manuel live in a country area and grow a great selection of vegetables, including salad vegetables through the summer months. They have free-range eggs from their hens, and a good, pure water system.

### General State of Health

Jean's stress levels had climbed above the normal for many reasons. At first, she felt irritable, hyperactive and distressed. She then began to have symptoms of bowel distress and menstrual cycle problems. Every morning when she rose from bed she would have diarrhea. She was referred to a specialist by her doctor. After a large number of tests, she was diagnosed as having a hyperactive thyroid gland, and she began treatment with a high dose of neo-mercazole. She began to respond after one month of this treatment.

### Symptoms

Some of the symptoms of hyperthyroidism, or thyrotoxicosis, are feeling too hot even when the temperature is cool; a great feeling of needing air, due to an increased need for oxygen by the body; heart palpitations or arrhythmia; excessive energy; poor sleep; and severe weight loss. It can affect men and women. In women, disturbance of the menstrual cycle can occur. Occasionally, there can be protrusion of the eyes.

Jean had symptoms of weight loss, heart rhythm irregularity, apprehension and anxiety as a result of her condition.

*Treatment Program*

Jean decided, with permission from her doctor, to work with a program of lifestyle and dietary adjustments, together with counseling. Studying Louise Hay's positive approaches to handling very difficult emotions became an important support throughout the program. Jean made an appointment to see the nutritional counselor.

On her first visit to her nutritionist, Jean made a list of very positive changes to her diet. Each day, she would include some organic grains, including millet, brown rice, whole oats, buckwheat, cornmeal, quinoa and wheat for whole-grain bread and pasta.

A special emphasis was placed on the following foods: adzuki beans; wax beans; dried fruit with sweet rice and millet; ginger; garlic; green vegetables (broccoli, kale, cabbage, sprouts); miso soup; protein drink (dairy-, egg-, sugar- and yeast-free); rice *or* buckwheat noodles; root vegetables (carrots, turnips, parsnips); and stewed fruit. The ginger and garlic were to improve the circulation and the appetite, and to calm the digestive system. Food supplements to help her digestion included acidophilus and kelp powder or tablets, in very small amounts. Special herbs were included in order to cleanse and heal the bowel, along with B-complex vitamins.

All the foods listed in Jean's menu have calming, centering, soothing and comforting properties. She consciously chose foods free from additives, residues or processing because her body would then not have to compete to receive its nutrients. She enjoyed her own eggs and made lots of salads in the summer. Fish and white meat were added to the diet as good sources of essential fats and protein.

*REBUILDING THE BODY*

Because Jean had lost a lot of weight, and consequently minerals, vitamins, enzymes and essential fats, it was absolutely vital to include top-quality supplements in her program. Jean became very intuitive about the needs of her own body. At her consultations, she discussed how she was feeling both physically and emotionally. She related how helpful she found the protein drink, which staved off the sinking feeling she used to have between meals. It also gave her sufficient energy to prepare her next meal.

Jean's requirements for essential fats (CFA) were very great. Her previous eating habits had not included sufficient sources. Now her hormonal and nervous systems were causing concern. Evening primrose oil was added to the program, in order to begin the process of healing. Fatty acids are the foundations and the protectors of a strong, healthy nervous system. Since folic acid and vitamin $B_{12}$ are two of the cooperating workers involved in the synthesis of essential fats, the evening primrose was taken at the same time as the protein drink, which contained both. As she became more skilled in the management of her shopping and preparation of foods, Jean tried new sources of essential fats, which also happened to be calcium- and magnesium-rich.

*NEW FOODS*

Jean then integrated a variety of new foods into her diet, including almonds (toasted and ground in a coffee grinder); dillisk *or* dulse *or* wakame (all rich sources of minerals, including calcium and iron, and also fats); feta cheese; sea vegetables, e.g. kombu (added to soups, casseroles and vegetable dishes); sunflower seeds; tahini (sesame seed spread); tofu; and vegetarian cheese.

*SAMPLE LUNCH MENU*

One pita bread, toasted to pop open, with various fillings including shredded lettuce, chopped chives, feta cheese, small tomato or a little red pepper, one teaspoon olive oil, chopped basil. Mix the filling together. Open up the pita bread, fill with mixture, decorate with watercress. In winter, a hot bowl of a soup such as minute soup to begin the meal; in summer natural yogurt after the meal.

A recipe for minute soup is as follows. Liquefy one mug of lightly cooked carrots and one mug of cooked, diced potatoes. Add two mugs of vegetable juice from previously cooked vegetables *or* add pure unsweetened carrot juice. Heat through — do not boil. Decorate with parsley and sage.

## COUNSELING

During the year, Jean began to receive counseling, which she found of immense help in settling her emotions. Her priorities gradually changed from very high expectations of perfection to more achievable goals. Belief systems she had held for a long time were revealed and replaced with new, positive thought patterns.

## OUTCOME

The effects of the chosen foods could be seen over the next few months. Jean gradually found herself becoming less overwhelmed, less impatient, less tense and hyperactive. She also noticed herself being more and more satisfied with her meals, and correctly concluded that this was due to the increasing efficiency of her digestion.

Jean also began a course in theater development. This included learning to discover the child within. This was a turning point in her life, and Jean's happiness was wonderful to see. Her eyes had a new light, her appetite improved and she began to put back on the lost weight. All diarrhea stopped. Her menstrual cycle became normal, and her nervous system became calm. Now she wanted to achieve her greatest desire — to have a child.

Her specialist reduced the neo-mercazole very slowly to the minimum dose. Her nutrition was changed to pre-pregnancy vitamins and minerals and folic acid. Within six weeks, the happy news was that Jean and Manuel were expecting their first child. Jean's health was exceptional throughout the pregnancy. Their baby girl arrived safe and sound. It can be said that due — at least in part — to the wonderful nutritional regime followed by both parents (Manuel ate the same food as Jean), the baby had a gentle, swift entry into the world.

The baby is healthy, calm and good-humored. Needless to say, Jean is extremely pleased with her new way of eating. She feels it was worth all the effort she made at the very start of her program to become a skilled cook of natural, whole, unprocessed foods. The benefits are to be seen in each family member.

## CASE THREE: MARK

Twelve-year-old Mark was referred to me for kinesiology, allergy tests and nutrition by a remarkable priest who also has the gift of healing. The priest felt that Mark was in need not only of spiritual but also of nutritional help. Mark's case illustrates very well the way holistic healing recognizes that the person is a spiritual as well as physical being, and that all the individual's aspects — mental, emotional and physical — may need to be addressed in the process of healing. Mark's ambition was to be a top-class athlete, although his lack of energy was severely restricting the amount of soccer and other games he could play.

### DIET

Mark's diet was high in dairy foods.

### GENERAL STATE OF HEALTH

Mark was underweight for his age, completely lacking in energy and suffering from severe bouts of asthma. He was missing a lot of school and was emotionally upset at times. There was no family history of any degenerative disease — although previous generations experienced poor circulation and respiratory problems — and until recently there had been no cancer in the family. His parents, strong people who had previously both been well, were suffering from stress and general ill health.

## KINESIOLOGY AND NUTRITIONAL TESTS

The kinesiology tests showed Mark to be living in a house with high levels of electromagnetic energy and geopathic stress (i.e. water under the ground that disturbs the function of the human body). Both can be caused by electrical equipment, such as microwaves, pylons outside the home, underground water and radon gas.

The nutritional tests found that Mark was very undernourished due to a weak and poorly functioning thyroid gland which in turn affected his metabolism. This was the cause of his sluggishness and the fact that he felt cold even in warm rooms. His allergy test showed that certain foods he was regularly eating were not agreeing with him and were causing good foods to be blocked in their absorption.

The highest allergy foods were all dairy products, yeast, beet sugar, monosodium glutamate, additives, chemicals, colorings and preservatives. All of these can be triggers for hyperactive behavior, asthma, urticaria, gastric stomach, insomnia and vomiting.

## TREATMENT PROGRAM

We discussed the environment, the allergies and a new dietary approach that would, over the next two months, exclude the known allergic foods.

Mark's parents were advised to switch off as much of their electrical equipment as possible and to allow a very limited amount of television. Other measures included moving Mark into a spare bedroom that was farther away from electrical equipment such as fuse boxes, video recorders and the television; children are more sensitive to electromagnetic waves than adults.

Mark's nutritional program included a gradual move onto goat's milk, yogurt and cheese. Extra supplies of foods that benefit the respiratory system had to be included in Mark's diet, such as chicken broth (contains an anti-inflammatory); garlic; green vegetable soups; homemade barley and lemon water; lemons; lentil, chickpea *or* split pea soup. A good, nourishing, hot breakfast every morning was important — whole-grain bread, oatmeal, homemade pancakes, scrambled eggs on toast, potatoes and rice made into burger or sausage shapes and grilled or fried in good-quality oil, potato cakes with spaghetti made from buckwheat, corn or rice.

For lunch, Mark was to have hot soup, a salad and sandwich made with rye, oat or whole-grain bread. Dinner was to include two vegetables (one green); whole-grain rice, buckwheat, corn *or* millet *or* potato; with one of the following: chicken, fish, lamb, turkey, vegetarian risotto, vegetarian *or* lamb lasagne *or* vegetable casserole. For dessert, Mark was to eat homemade apple pie, apple *or* rhubarb crumble, apple strudel, natural yogurt.

It was important to add lots of parsley, onion, garlic, thyme and horseradish to the foods. Liquids included hot lemon, barley and honey drinks, to clear the mucous congestion from the respiratory system. Recommended supplements were

- aromatherapy oil of eucalyptus in a very high dilution, with almond oil (for massaging the chest and lungs every morning and evening)

- Bach flower remedies (specially chosen to strengthen, encourage and motivate Mark to get better)

- cod liver oil

- evening primrose oil

- garlic capsules

- vitamin C (buffered, i.e. non-acid, which is more easily tolerated by delicate stomachs)

## OUTCOME

Over a period of two months, the treatment program brought about a remarkable degree of recovery, and Mark is still in touch two years later. He is continuing to go from strength to strength. Mark's mother had his complete cooperation from the very outset of his treatment; she explained everything about his diet and lifestyle that she was changing, and asked him for feedback. His appetite became good, he enjoyed all his food and was willing to try new dishes. He gained weight, slept very well, and was able to fight off any threat of a cold, cough or infection that might start up the asthma again. Mark has also noticed a greater tolerance of weather changes. His doctor has monitored his doses of asthma medicine throughout, gradually reducing the prescription as needed.

Finally, Mark is progressing very well in physical sports, particularly soccer.

## FURTHER RECOMMENDATIONS

In winter, the elderberry fruit was recommended as a regular part of Mark's prevention regime. Made into a hot drink with peppermint tea and honey, it acts against inflammation of the mucous membranes; it is also rich in vitamin C — and it is in any case delicious! Suggestions that have proven helpful in the steady and continuing healing of Mark's lungs have been reflexology, deep breathing exercises and maintaining a good posture. Good posture was emphasized because those with lung problems tend to hunch their shoulders and develop a round shoulder posture, which is very unhealthy.

## CASE FOUR: ROBERT

Robert, a five-year-old boy with Down's syndrome, came to see me, brought by his mother.

### DIET

Robert's favorite foods, of which he ate a lot, were sweet rolls and cookies, cheddar cheese sandwiches, and ice cream.

### GENERAL STATE OF HEALTH

Robert's biggest problem is his susceptibility to colds, which go straight down to his chest, becoming a constant cough that nothing seems to clear. He also produces a mucous discharge from his nose.

### TREATMENT PROGRAM

Robert's mother and I discussed at length how best to rearrange his diet, in order to incorporate less of the above foods and more fruit and vegetables. We agreed that she would slowly, over a period of two months, make the necessary changes to Robert's diet.

My suggestions were as follows: for breakfast three mornings a week, Robert was to have baby oat flakes porridge with honey and a little milk; two mornings a week, he was to have a high-fiber, low-sugar (raw sugar) cereal, with juice or milk; on the remaining two mornings, he would have an egg or beans on brown, whole-grain toast.

Mid-morning, Robert could have fresh fruit in season and a drink of water. Lunch would consist of a bowl of carrot and potato soup *or* chicken broth *or* vegetable soup (mainly green vegetables, with added parsley and onions) *or* lentil soup, with whole-grain brown bread scones *or* rice cakes *or* rye bread *or* oat cakes with tahini spread *or* almond nut butter *or* sunflower butter.

His mid-afternoon snack would be fresh fruit in season (e.g. mashed banana) with a dairy-free ice cream, such as soy ice cream. For dinner, Robert could have a puréed (instead of chopped) selection of vegetables; with potatoes, rice *or* whole grain pasta; and fish, turkey, chicken *or* lamb; dessert was to be natural yogurt and a slice of carrot cake. (Vegetable purée is far more easily digested and a more valuable source of nutrition for children.)

### ADDITIONAL SUGGESTIONS

A selection of Bach flower remedies were made up to help Robert to adjust to the dietary changes and to strengthen his immune system. The aromatherapy oils chamomile and lavender were made up in almond oil to massage the little boy's back and chest twice daily, in order to increase circulation, strengthen the lung muscles and build up resistance to infection. The oils were greatly diluted because of Robert's age.

I also suggested that Robert spend less time sitting in front of the television, with instead more walks and sports. I emphasized that small meals were sensible, since little and often at the age of five is very helpful to the developing digestive system and helps the child avoid obesity.

### OUTCOME

I have kept in touch with Robert and his mother for over six years. He has become a fine, radiantly healthy young boy who enjoys his food, school, his friends and family.

## CASE FIVE: MAEVE

Maeve is a woman who found difficulty in achieving correct diagnosis or assistance through conventional medical treatment. Her mother's protracted illness and subsequent death had put Maeve under considerable stress. Following conventional treatment for problems with her uterus, Maeve found out about alternative medicine, which she decided to try.

## GENERAL STATE OF HEALTH

Maeve had three small operations on her uterus in 1994, which needed subsequent treatment with two courses of antibiotics. Her immune system was low, and she had a viral flu that left her so tired she spent ten days able to do nothing but sit on the couch. On a visit to her physician she was told that nothing could be done for her, and that her exhaustion may have been from Chronic Fatigue Syndrome, a common aftermath of viral flu.

## SYMPTOMS

Along with the extreme tiredness, Maeve has a number of other problems. Her stomach and bowel swell up after eating certain foods, and this is accompanied by an uncomfortable, itchy feeling. She has a craving for sweet foods and chocolate, and eating sugar in any food causes her skin to break out in a rash, especially on her back. Her sinuses are also irritated; she becomes breathless just walking up the stairs and has no energy. Consequently, her mental state is one of complete despondency.

## KINESIOLOGY AND VEGA TESTS

Maeve underwent Vega testing. This measures the bio-energy in the body and delivers bio-information produced by the internal organs and systems. It is based on measuring electrical conductivity by applying an electrode, which is held by the patient.

These tests revealed that Maeve had *Candida albicans* — a yeast infection; she had an intolerance to sugar and yeast; her immune system was very low; her liver and small intestine were affected; and she had a chemical allergy. Maeve was very relieved to discover what the root cause of her problem was.

### Treatment Program

Maeve immediately began an anti-candida program, cutting out all sugar and yeast from her diet and using supplements. She also used homeopathic anti-fungal drops. After six weeks, she introduced caprylic acid, which kills off the candida infection in the body. The reaction to the treatment meant that Maeve felt somewhat worse for a few weeks, with flu-like symptoms and pains in her legs.

### Short-Term Outcome

Having completed this stage of the treatment, Maeve felt much better, even though she had lost a lot of weight.

### Additional Dietary Measures

Maeve then began to eat garlic, and took cold-pressed virgin olive oil. She also took the herbal tea pau d'arco, which is anti-fungal, and drank aloe vera juice. She began to replace the friendly bacteria in the bowel with a course of acidophilus. She discovered a wonderful herb, goldenseal, which is anti-fungal, antibiotic and in addition boosts the immune system.

### A Setback

Maeve felt so much better after six months, although still much thinner than she had been before, that she celebrated her new-found energy and health with two vodkas. However, because of her sensitivity to chemicals, this set her back considerably. Having put a strain on her liver with the chemical overload, her intestinal ecology was upset, which encouraged the parasites. Maeve was then treated with grapefruit seed extract. Because her body was not breaking down foods into usable nutrients, she was put on digestive enzymes.

## LONG-TERM OUTCOME

It took eighteen months in total for the candida to be cleared out of Maeve's system. She is still careful with her diet and her alcohol intake. It has been a tremendous learning experience for her, and she believes that the over-use of antibiotics and the over-consumption of processed foods are bringing about increasing numbers of cases of candida. Maeve is doing very well, and has begun studying anatomy, physiology and nutrition, with a view toward a degree.

# APPENDIX ONE

---

## HERBS AND THEIR BENEFITS

| *Herb* | *Benefits* |
| --- | --- |
| Almond | Skin |
| Aloe vera | Skin |
| Anise | Digestion |
| Apple | Digestion, lowers cholesterol |
| Artichoke | Liver |
| Basil | Digestion |
| Blueberry | Eyesight |
| Borage | Gamma linoleic acid |
| Calendula | Pain reliever |
| Chamomile | Vitamin C |
| Capsicum | Vitamin C |
| Caraway | Digestion |

| | |
|---|---|
| Carrot | Anti-cancer |
| Cayenne | Soothing |
| Comfrey | Relieves sores |
| Cranberry | Liver, gallbladder |
| Dandelion | Boosts immune system |
| Echinacea | Anti-urinary tract infection |
| Evening primrose | Reduces stress and tension |
| Fenugreek | Lowers blood sugar levels |
| Feverfew | Headaches |
| Garlic | Antibiotic effect, anti-cancer |
| Ginger | Digestion, calms stomach |
| Ginkgo | All-round booster |
| Ginseng | Increases endurance |
| Golden seal | Skin problems |
| Horse chestnut | Veins |
| Juniper berry | Urinary tract infections |
| Nettle | Lowers blood sugar, iron |
| Raspberry | Good for women generally |
| Shiitake mushroom | Boosts immune system |
| Turmeric | Cleans blood, gallbladder |

## FOODS AND THEIR PROPERTIES

| Foods | Properties |
|---|---|
| Garlic, onions, raw carrots, shiitake mushrooms | Anti-cancer |
| Turmeric, garlic, cayenne and ginkgo | Circulation |

| | |
|---|---|
| Evening primrose, cayenne, garlic, olive oil, oat bran, artichoke | Heart |
| Echinacea | Immune system booster |
| Milk thistle, artichoke, dandelion, turmeric | Liver |

## FOOD SOURCES OF MINERALS

| *Mineral* | *Sources* |
|---|---|
| Phosphorus | Alfalfa, avocado, beets, Brussels sprouts, cabbage, coconut, corn, peas |
| Potassium | Alfalfa, avocado, beans (green), dates, dandelions, greens, parsnips, potato peel |
| Silicon | Beets, cantaloupe, grains (whole, sprouted), horseradish, horsetail and oat straw tea, parsnips |
| Sodium | Alfalfa, cabbage, carrots, celery, goat's milk (and whey), lettuce, spinach, watermelon |
| Sulphur | Alfalfa, avocado, Brussels sprouts, broccoli, cabbage, cranberries, kale, pumpkin, watercress |

## BOTANICAL VITAMIN SOURCES

| *Vitamin* | *Sources* |
|---|---|
| Vitamin A | Alfalfa, annatto, dandelion, watercress, parsley, paprika, kelp |

| | |
|---|---|
| Vitamin B | Apples, bananas, beans, beets, cabbage, carrots, corn, grapefruit, onions, oranges, peas, potatoes, raisins, spinach, tomatoes, wheat, whole seeds, yeast |
| Vitamin C complex | All greens and citrus fruits |
| Vitamin C | Annatto, watercress, wheat germ, all oil-containing seeds |
| Vitamin D | All seeds, alfalfa, oats, flax, sesame, wheat germ, soybeans, tofu, dulse, kelp, watercress |
| Vitamin E | Alfalfa, chestnut leaves |
| Vitamin K | Rose hips, black and red currants, strawberries, potatoes, spinach, cabbage, watercress |

## FOODS FOR RAPID HEALING

| | |
|---|---|
| *Fruits* | Apples, apricots, cherries, dates, figs (fresh or dried), grapefruit, grapes, lemons, oranges, peaches, pears, plums, prunes (dried), raisins, raspberries and strawberries |
| *Vegetables* | Asparagus, beans (green), cabbage (raw), carrots (raw), cauliflower (raw), celery (raw), cucumber, garlic, green peppers, lettuce, onions (raw), parsnips, peas, spinach, tomatoes and watercress |

# APPENDIX TWO:
# A TYPICAL DAILY
# MENU

---

This menu is based on the principle of restoring health; the ingredients have been chosen to stimulate your metabolism, nourish the muscles, and help you stabilize your weight.

*Breakfast*  Swiss muesli based on oat flakes or millet flakes, with chopped apricots (steeped overnight in water) *or* almonds *or* a little pear, apple *or* berries, blueberries, blackberries, blackcurrants; tea (low caffeine); whole-grain rye *or* wheat bread; almond *or* tahini spread; sugar-free marmalade *or* sugar-free fruit jam.

*Lunch*  Vegetable soup *or* homemade soup made from any meat, *or* some chicken *or* fish; baked potato with coleslaw *or* cottage cheese with herbs (parsley, watercress, horseradish, garlic); a small salad in winter, a large salad in summer, including as many available grains and vegetables as you like.

*Dinner* Try to eat an early meal, with plenty of time to enjoy and digest it before retiring. Eat traditional dishes such as casserole of vegetables and meat, with lentils, chickpeas or adzuki beans. If you plan ahead, you can cook enough grain for three days. Combine rice, millet or whole grain pasta with a tasty selection of vegetables. Add any meat or fish in a very small amount, with soup.

*Suggested dinner menu* Vegetarian *or* meat lasagne. If you make meat lasagne, halve the meat content by using an equal quantity of red lentils, pre-cooked for twenty minutes (one cup of lentils to two cups water or stock).

Vegetarian curry *or* meat curry. Reduce the meat by including extra vegetables *or* chickpeas.

Vegetarian nut loaf *or* meat loaf. Again, reduce the quantity of meat by adding one cup of cooked grains.

Stir-fry dish. Try a potato and vegetable selection; simply cut your vegetables up into similar-sized chunks, including the potatoes. Cook potato and onion in olive *or* sunflower oil for six to eight minutes, then add diced red pepper and carrots. Cook for about three minutes until crunchy, then add tomatoes, garlic, parsley, feta cheese, tofu, chicken *or* fish. Put a lid on your wok or saucepan. Heat through thoroughly, and serve with salad, rice noodles, whole-grain spaghetti *or* millet. The total preparation and cooking time is only around twenty-five minutes or less.

# RECOMMENDED READING

Airola, Paavo O., *Health Secrets from Europe* (Arco Publishing, 1972)

Barnard, Julian and Martine, *The Healing Herbs of Edward Bach* (Ashgrove Press Limited, 1997)

Bircher Benner Clinic, *Bircher Benner Nutrition Plan for Skin Problems* (Pyramid Books, 1973)

Carson, Rachel, *Silent Spring* (Houghton-Mifflin Company, 1963)

Chelminski, Rudolph, "A Great Way to Live Longer," in *Reader's Digest*, September 1994

Clark, Hulda Regehr, *The Cure for All Cancers* (New Century Press, 1993)

Clark, Hulda Regehr, *The Cure for All Diseases* (New Century Press, 1995)

Colbin, Annemarie, *Food and Healing* (Ballantine Books, 1986)

Davies, Steven and Stewart, Alan, *A Nutritional Medicine* (Pan Books, 1987)

De Vries, Jan, *Menopause* (Mainstream Press, 1993)

De Vries, Jan, *Menstrual and Premenstrual Tension* (Trafalgar, 1992)

De Vries, Jan, *Stress and Nervous Disorders* (Mainstream Press, 1994)

Emsley, John, *The Consumer's Good Chemical Guide* (Corgi, 1996)

Fathman, George and Doris, *Live Foods* (Ehret Literature Publishing, 1967)

Flatto, Edwin, *Revitalize Your Body with Nature's Secrets* (Arco Publishing, 1973)

Grieve, M., *A Modern Herbal* (Dover Publications, 1978)

Halvorsen, Brian and Flemming, Susan, *The Natural Dentist* (Century Arrow, 1986)

Hay, Louise, *Empowering Women* (Hay House, 1997)

Heinerman, John, *Heinerman's Encyclopedia of Fruits and Vegetables* (Parker, 1995)

Katz, Martha Ellen, *High Protein Baking* (Ballantine, 1975)

Kiester, Edwin and Valente, Sally, "Little Known Signs of a Heart Attack," in *Reader's Digest*, August 1993

Kinderlehrer, Jane, *How to Feel Younger Longer* (Rodale, 1974)

Lacey, Richard, *Unfit for Human Consumption, Food in Crisis* (Grafton, 1991)

Lappe, Frances Moore, *Diet for a Small Planet* (Ballantine, 1991)

Larson, Gena, *Better Food for Better Babies and Their Families* (Keats Publishing, 1980)

Mansfield, Peter and Monro, Jean, *Chemical Children* (Century, 1987)

Mayes, Kathleen, *Brittle Bone and Osteoporosis — The Calcium Crisis* (Grapevine, 1987)

Miller, Saul and Miller, Jo Anne, *Food for Thought* (Prentice Hall, 1979)

Mindell, Earl, *The Vitamin Bible* (Warner Books, 1991)

Mindell, Earl, *The Vitamin Bible for Your Children* (Arlington Books, 1981)

Nambudripad, Devi S., *Say Goodbye to Illness* (Pain Clinic, 1993)

Pekkanen, John, "Seven Health Symptoms You Must Not Ignore," in *Reader's Digest*, October 1992

*Permaculture Magazine*, Permanent Publications

Pitchford, Paul, *Healing with Whole Foods: Oriental Traditions and Modern Nutrition* (North Atlantic Books, 1996)

Poesnecker, G. E., *Adrenal Syndrome, The Disease No Doctor Wants to Treat* (Humanitarian Publishing, 1983)

Price, Weston, *Nutrition and Physical Degeneration* (Keats Publishing, 1997)

Rapp, Doris J., *Allergies and Your Family* (Sterling Publications, 1981)

Rogers, Sherry A., *Tired or Toxic?* (Prestige, 1990)

Sheinkin, David, Schachter, Michael and Hutton, Richard, *Food — Mind and Mood* (Warner Books, 1979)

Smith, Lendon, *Feed Your Kids Right* (Dell Publishing, 1988)

Trattler, Ross, *Better Health through Natural Healing: How to Get Well without Drugs or Surgery* (Thorson's, 1987)

Vogel, Alfred, *The Nature Doctor* (Keats Publishing, 1991)

Wade, Carlson, *Helping Your Health with Enzymes* (Arco Publishing, 1966)

Wade, Carlson, *Magic Minerals* (Arco Publishing, 1967)

Weeks, Nora, *The Medical Discoveries of Dr. Bach* (Keats Publishing, 1994)

Weil, Andrew, *Spontaneous Healing* (Knopf, 1995)

**FURTHER READING**

Chopra, Deepak, *Perfect Health* (Harmony Books, 1991)

Chopra, Deepak, *Quantum Healing* (Bantam, 1986)

Hoffman, David, *New Holistic Herbal* (Element Books, 1991)

Lewis, Alan, *The Natural Athlete* (Century, 1984)

Scott, Julian, *Natural Medicine for Children* (Avon Books, 1996)

Sinha, Phulgenda, *Yogic Cure for Common Ailments* (Ind-Us, 1981)

# INDEX

# ULYSSES PRESS HEALTH BOOKS

## DISCOVER HANDBOOKS

Easy to follow and authoritative, *Discover Handbooks* reveal an array of alternative therapies from around the world and demonstrate how to incorporate them into a program of good health.

Each book opens with information on the history and principles of the particular technique, then presents practical and straightforward guidance on ways in which it can be applied. Offering the tools needed to achieve and maintain an optimal state of health, the approach is one of personal improvement and self-reliance. Each of the books features: an introduction to the discipline; an explanation of its philosophy; step-by-step guide to its implementation; clear diagrams and charts; and case studies.

DISCOVER AYURVEDA
ISBN 1-56975-081-5, 128 pp, $8.95

DISCOVER COLOR THERAPY
ISBN 1-56975-093-9, 144 pp, $8.95

DISCOVER ESSENTIAL OILS
ISBN 1-56975-080-7, 128 pp, $8.95

DISCOVER MEDITATION
ISBN 1-56975-113-7, 144 pp, $8.95

DISCOVER NUTRITIONAL THERAPY
ISBN 1-56975-135-8, 120 pp, $8.95

DISCOVER OSTEOPATHY
ISBN 1-56975-115-3, 132 pp, $8.95

DISCOVER REFLEXOLOGY
ISBN 1-56975-112-9, 132 pp, $8.95

DISCOVER SHIATSU
ISBN 1-56975-082-3, 128 pp, $8.95

## THE ANCIENT AND HEALING ARTS BOOKS

*The Ancient and Healing Arts* books recount the development of healing art forms that have been used for thousands of years. Beautifully illustrated with full color on every page, they discuss the benefits of these time-honored techniques and offer detailed instructions on their use.

THE ANCIENT AND HEALING ART OF AROMATHERAPY
ISBN 1-56975-094-7, 96 pp, $14.95

THE ANCIENT AND HEALING ART OF CHINESE HERBALISM
ISBN 1-56975-139-0, 96 pp, $14.95

# NATURAL APPROACH BOOKS

Written in a friendly, nontechnical style, *A Natural Approach* books address specific health issues and show you how to take an active part in your own treatment. Whether you suffer from panic attacks, endometriosis or depression, each book will provide you with a thorough understanding of your condition and detail organic solutions that offer immediate relief for your symptoms and effectively remedy their underlying causes.

Believing that disease is more than a combination of symptoms, these books offer integrated mind/body programs that take a positive, preventative approach. Since traditional drug therapy is not always the best solution (and can sometimes be the problem), these guides show how to use alternative treatments to supplement or replace conventional medicine.

ANXIETY & DEPRESSION
ISBN 1-56975-118-8, 144 pp, $9.95

IRRITABLE BOWEL SYNDROME
ISBN 1-56975-030-0, 240 pp, $11.95

ENDOMETRIOSIS
ISBN 1-56975-088-2, 184 pp, 9.95

MIGRAINES
ISBN 1-56975-140-4, 156 pp, $8.95

FREE YOURSELF FROM TRANQUILIZERS
& SLEEPING PILLS
ISBN 1-56975-074-2, 192 pp, $9.95

PANIC ATTACKS
ISBN 1-56975-045-9, 148 pp, $9.95

IRRITABLE BLADDER & INCONTINENCE
ISBN 1-56975-089-0, 108 pp, $8.95

# THE NATURAL REMEDY BOOKS

As home remedies and alternative treatments become increasingly accepted into the medical mainstream, people want information—not just hype and unproven claims—about the remedies they see in health food stores. *The Natural Remedy* books detail how these natural remedies have been used throughout history and how to safely incorporate them into an overall plan for maintaining good health.

CIDER VINEGAR
ISBN 1-56975-141-2, 144 pp, $8.95

GARLIC
ISBN 1-56975-097-1, 152 pp, $9.95

# OTHER HEALTH TITLES

THE BOOK OF KOMBUCHA
ISBN 1-56975-049-1, 160 pp, $11.95
Explains the benefits of and addresses concerns about Kombucha, the widely used Chinese "tea mushroom."

HEALING REIKI: REUNITE MIND, BODY AND SPIRIT
WITH HEALING ENERGIES
ISBN 1-56975-162-5, 124 pp, $16.95
Examines the meaning, perception and history of this ancient healing technique while providing practical tips for giving and receiving Reiki.

HEPATITIS C: A PERSONAL GUIDE TO GOOD HEALTH
ISBN 1-56975-091-2, 172 pp, $12.95
Identifies the causes and symptoms of hepatitis C and presents conventional and alternative treatments for coping with the disease.

KNOW YOUR BODY: THE ATLAS OF ANATOMY
ISBN 1-56975-021-1, 160 pp, $12.95
Presents a full-color guide to the structure of the human body.

MOOD FOODS
ISBN 1-56975-023-8, 192 pp, $9.95
Shows how the foods you eat influence your emotions and behavior.

YOUR NATURAL PREGNANCY: A GUIDE TO COMPLEMENTARY THERAPIES
ISBN 1-56975-059-9, 240 pp, $16.95
Details alternative therapies ranging from aromatherapy to yoga that can benefit pregnant women.

---

*To order these books call 800-377-2542, e-mail ulysses@ulyssespress.com, fax 510-601-8307 or write to Ulysses Press, P.O. Box 3440, Berkeley, CA 94703. All retail orders are shipped free of charge. California residents must include sales Allow two to three weeks for delivery.*